Synaesthesia: A Very Short Introduction

VERY SHORT INTRODUCTIONS are for anyone wanting a stimulating and accessible way into a new subject. They are written by experts, and have been translated into more than 45 different languages.

The series began in 1995, and now covers a wide variety of topics in every discipline. The VSI library currently contains over 600 volumes—a Very Short Introduction to everything from Psychology and Philosophy of Science to American History and Relativity—and continues to grow in every subject area.

Very Short Introductions available now:

ABOLITIONISM Richard S. Newman
ACCOUNTING Christopher Nobes
ADAM SMITH Christopher J. Berry
ADOLESCENCE Peter K. Smith
ADVERTISING Winston Fletcher
AFRICAN AMERICAN
    RELIGION Eddie S. Glaude Jr
AFRICAN HISTORY John Parker and
    Richard Rathbone
AFRICAN POLITICS Ian Taylor
AFRICAN RELIGIONS
    Jacob K. Olupona
AGEING Nancy A. Pachana
AGNOSTICISM Robin Le Poidevin
AGRICULTURE Paul Brassley and
    Richard Soffe
ALEXANDER THE GREAT
    Hugh Bowden
ALGEBRA Peter M. Higgins
AMERICAN CULTURAL HISTORY
    Eric Avila
AMERICAN FOREIGN RELATIONS
    Andrew Preston
AMERICAN HISTORY Paul S. Boyer
AMERICAN IMMIGRATION
    David A. Gerber
AMERICAN LEGAL HISTORY
    G. Edward White
AMERICAN NAVAL HISTORY
    Craig L. Symonds
AMERICAN POLITICAL HISTORY
    Donald Critchlow
AMERICAN POLITICAL PARTIES
    AND ELECTIONS L. Sandy Maisel

AMERICAN POLITICS
    Richard M. Valelly
THE AMERICAN PRESIDENCY
    Charles O. Jones
THE AMERICAN REVOLUTION
    Robert J. Allison
AMERICAN SLAVERY
    Heather Andrea Williams
THE AMERICAN WEST Stephen Aron
AMERICAN WOMEN'S HISTORY
    Susan Ware
ANAESTHESIA Aidan O'Donnell
ANALYTIC PHILOSOPHY
    Michael Beaney
ANARCHISM Colin Ward
ANCIENT ASSYRIA Karen Radner
ANCIENT EGYPT Ian Shaw
ANCIENT EGYPTIAN ART AND
    ARCHITECTURE Christina Riggs
ANCIENT GREECE Paul Cartledge
THE ANCIENT NEAR EAST
    Amanda H. Podany
ANCIENT PHILOSOPHY Julia Annas
ANCIENT WARFARE Harry Sidebottom
ANGELS David Albert Jones
ANGLICANISM Mark Chapman
THE ANGLO-SAXON AGE John Blair
ANIMAL BEHAVIOUR
    Tristram D. Wyatt
THE ANIMAL KINGDOM
    Peter Holland
ANIMAL RIGHTS David DeGrazia
THE ANTARCTIC Klaus Dodds
ANTHROPOCENE Erle C. Ellis

ANTISEMITISM Steven Beller
ANXIETY Daniel Freeman and
    Jason Freeman
THE APOCRYPHAL GOSPELS
    Paul Foster
APPLIED MATHEMATICS Alain Goriely
ARCHAEOLOGY Paul Bahn
ARCHITECTURE Andrew Ballantyne
ARISTOCRACY William Doyle
ARISTOTLE Jonathan Barnes
ART HISTORY Dana Arnold
ART THEORY Cynthia Freeland
ARTIFICIAL INTELLIGENCE
    Margaret A. Boden
ASIAN AMERICAN HISTORY
    Madeline Y. Hsu
ASTROBIOLOGY David C. Catling
ASTROPHYSICS James Binney
ATHEISM Julian Baggini
THE ATMOSPHERE Paul I. Palmer
AUGUSTINE Henry Chadwick
AUSTRALIA Kenneth Morgan
AUTISM Uta Frith
AUTOBIOGRAPHY Laura Marcus
THE AVANT GARDE David Cottington
THE AZTECS David Carrasco
BABYLONIA Trevor Bryce
BACTERIA Sebastian G. B. Amyes
BANKING John Goddard and
    John O. S. Wilson
BARTHES Jonathan Culler
THE BEATS David Sterritt
BEAUTY Roger Scruton
BEHAVIOURAL ECONOMICS
    Michelle Baddeley
BESTSELLERS John Sutherland
THE BIBLE John Riches
BIBLICAL ARCHAEOLOGY
    Eric H. Cline
BIG DATA Dawn E. Holmes
BIOGRAPHY Hermione Lee
BIOMETRICS Michael Fairhurst
BLACK HOLES Katherine Blundell
BLOOD Chris Cooper
THE BLUES Elijah Wald
THE BODY Chris Shilling
THE BOOK OF COMMON
    PRAYER Brian Cummings
THE BOOK OF MORMON
    Terryl Givens

BORDERS Alexander C. Diener and
    Joshua Hagen
THE BRAIN Michael O'Shea
BRANDING Robert Jones
THE BRICS Andrew F. Cooper
THE BRITISH CONSTITUTION
    Martin Loughlin
THE BRITISH EMPIRE Ashley Jackson
BRITISH POLITICS Anthony Wright
BUDDHA Michael Carrithers
BUDDHISM Damien Keown
BUDDHIST ETHICS Damien Keown
BYZANTIUM Peter Sarris
C. S. LEWIS James Como
CALVINISM Jon Balserak
CANCER Nicholas James
CAPITALISM James Fulcher
CATHOLICISM Gerald O'Collins
CAUSATION Stephen Mumford and
    Rani Lill Anjum
THE CELL Terence Allen and
    Graham Cowling
THE CELTS Barry Cunliffe
CHAOS Leonard Smith
CHARLES DICKENS Jenny Hartley
CHEMISTRY Peter Atkins
CHILD PSYCHOLOGY Usha Goswami
CHILDREN'S LITERATURE
    Kimberley Reynolds
CHINESE LITERATURE Sabina Knight
CHOICE THEORY Michael Allingham
CHRISTIAN ART Beth Williamson
CHRISTIAN ETHICS D. Stephen Long
CHRISTIANITY Linda Woodhead
CIRCADIAN RHYTHMS
    Russell Foster and Leon Kreitzman
CITIZENSHIP Richard Bellamy
CIVIL ENGINEERING
    David Muir Wood
CLASSICAL LITERATURE William Allan
CLASSICAL MYTHOLOGY
    Helen Morales
CLASSICS Mary Beard and
    John Henderson
CLAUSEWITZ Michael Howard
CLIMATE Mark Maslin
CLIMATE CHANGE Mark Maslin
CLINICAL PSYCHOLOGY
    Susan Llewelyn and
    Katie Aafjes-van Doorn

COGNITIVE NEUROSCIENCE
Richard Passingham
THE COLD WAR Robert McMahon
COLONIAL AMERICA Alan Taylor
COLONIAL LATIN AMERICAN
LITERATURE Rolena Adorno
COMBINATORICS Robin Wilson
COMEDY Matthew Bevis
COMMUNISM Leslie Holmes
COMPARATIVE LITERATURE
Ben Hutchinson
COMPLEXITY John H. Holland
THE COMPUTER Darrel Ince
COMPUTER SCIENCE
Subrata Dasgupta
CONCENTRATION CAMPS
Dan Stone
CONFUCIANISM Daniel K. Gardner
THE CONQUISTADORS
Matthew Restall and
Felipe Fernández-Armesto
CONSCIENCE Paul Strohm
CONSCIOUSNESS Susan Blackmore
CONTEMPORARY ART
Julian Stallabrass
CONTEMPORARY FICTION
Robert Eaglestone
CONTINENTAL PHILOSOPHY
Simon Critchley
COPERNICUS Owen Gingerich
CORAL REEFS Charles Sheppard
CORPORATE SOCIAL
RESPONSIBILITY Jeremy Moon
CORRUPTION Leslie Holmes
COSMOLOGY Peter Coles
CRIME FICTION Richard Bradford
CRIMINAL JUSTICE Julian V. Roberts
CRIMINOLOGY Tim Newburn
CRITICAL THEORY
Stephen Eric Bronner
THE CRUSADES Christopher Tyerman
CRYPTOGRAPHY Fred Piper and
Sean Murphy
CRYSTALLOGRAPHY A. M. Glazer
THE CULTURAL REVOLUTION
Richard Curt Kraus
DADA AND SURREALISM
David Hopkins
DANTE Peter Hainsworth and
David Robey
DARWIN Jonathan Howard

THE DEAD SEA SCROLLS
Timothy H. Lim
DECADENCE David Weir
DECOLONIZATION Dane Kennedy
DEMOCRACY Bernard Crick
DEMOGRAPHY Sarah Harper
DEPRESSION Jan Scott and
Mary Jane Tacchi
DERRIDA Simon Glendinning
DESCARTES Tom Sorell
DESERTS Nick Middleton
DESIGN John Heskett
DEVELOPMENT Ian Goldin
DEVELOPMENTAL BIOLOGY
Lewis Wolpert
THE DEVIL Darren Oldridge
DIASPORA Kevin Kenny
DICTIONARIES Lynda Mugglestone
DINOSAURS David Norman
DIPLOMACY Joseph M. Siracusa
DOCUMENTARY FILM
Patricia Aufderheide
DREAMING J. Allan Hobson
DRUGS Les Iversen
DRUIDS Barry Cunliffe
DYSLEXIA Margaret J. Snowling
EARLY MUSIC Thomas Forrest Kelly
THE EARTH Martin Redfern
EARTH SYSTEM SCIENCE
Tim Lenton
ECONOMICS Partha Dasgupta
EDUCATION Gary Thomas
EGYPTIAN MYTH Geraldine Pinch
EIGHTEENTH-CENTURY
BRITAIN Paul Langford
THE ELEMENTS Philip Ball
EMOTION Dylan Evans
EMPIRE Stephen Howe
ENGELS Terrell Carver
ENGINEERING David Blockley
THE ENGLISH LANGUAGE
Simon Horobin
ENGLISH LITERATURE Jonathan Bate
THE ENLIGHTENMENT
John Robertson
ENTREPRENEURSHIP Paul Westhead
and Mike Wright
ENVIRONMENTAL ECONOMICS
Stephen Smith
ENVIRONMENTAL ETHICS
Robin Attfield

ENVIRONMENTAL LAW
    Elizabeth Fisher
ENVIRONMENTAL POLITICS
    Andrew Dobson
EPICUREANISM Catherine Wilson
EPIDEMIOLOGY Rodolfo Saracci
ETHICS Simon Blackburn
ETHNOMUSICOLOGY
    Timothy Rice
THE ETRUSCANS Christopher Smith
EUGENICS Philippa Levine
THE EUROPEAN UNION
    Simon Usherwood and John Pinder
EUROPEAN UNION LAW
    Anthony Arnull
EVOLUTION Brian and
    Deborah Charlesworth
EXISTENTIALISM Thomas Flynn
EXPLORATION Stewart A. Weaver
EXTINCTION Paul B. Wignall
THE EYE Michael Land
FAIRY TALE Marina Warner
FAMILY LAW Jonathan Herring
FASCISM Kevin Passmore
FASHION Rebecca Arnold
FEMINISM Margaret Walters
FILM Michael Wood
FILM MUSIC Kathryn Kalinak
FILM NOIR James Naremore
THE FIRST WORLD WAR
    Michael Howard
FOLK MUSIC Mark Slobin
FOOD John Krebs
FORENSIC PSYCHOLOGY
    David Canter
FORENSIC SCIENCE Jim Fraser
FORESTS Jaboury Ghazoul
FOSSILS Keith Thomson
FOUCAULT Gary Gutting
THE FOUNDING FATHERS
    R. B. Bernstein
FRACTALS Kenneth Falconer
FREE SPEECH Nigel Warburton
FREE WILL Thomas Pink
FREEMASONRY Andreas Önnerfors
FRENCH LITERATURE John D. Lyons
THE FRENCH REVOLUTION
    William Doyle
FREUD Anthony Storr
FUNDAMENTALISM Malise Ruthven
FUNGI Nicholas P. Money

THE FUTURE Jennifer M. Gidley
GALAXIES John Gribbin
GALILEO Stillman Drake
GAME THEORY Ken Binmore
GANDHI Bhikhu Parekh
GARDEN HISTORY Gordon Campbell
GENES Jonathan Slack
GENIUS Andrew Robinson
GENOMICS John Archibald
GEOGRAPHY John Matthews and
    David Herbert
GEOLOGY Jan Zalasiewicz
GEOPHYSICS William Lowrie
GEOPOLITICS Klaus Dodds
GERMAN LITERATURE
    Nicholas Boyle
GERMAN PHILOSOPHY
    Andrew Bowie
GLACIATION David J. A. Evans
GLOBAL CATASTROPHES
    Bill McGuire
GLOBAL ECONOMIC HISTORY
    Robert C. Allen
GLOBALIZATION Manfred Steger
GOD John Bowker
GOETHE Ritchie Robertson
THE GOTHIC Nick Groom
GOVERNANCE Mark Bevir
GRAVITY Timothy Clifton
THE GREAT DEPRESSION AND
    THE NEW DEAL Eric Rauchway
HABERMAS James Gordon Finlayson
THE HABSBURG EMPIRE
    Martyn Rady
HAPPINESS Daniel M. Haybron
THE HARLEM
    RENAISSANCE Cheryl A. Wall
THE HEBREW BIBLE AS
    LITERATURE Tod Linafelt
HEGEL Peter Singer
HEIDEGGER Michael Inwood
THE HELLENISTIC AGE
    Peter Thonemann
HEREDITY John Waller
HERMENEUTICS Jens Zimmermann
HERODOTUS Jennifer T. Roberts
HIEROGLYPHS Penelope Wilson
HINDUISM Kim Knott
HISTORY John H. Arnold
THE HISTORY OF ASTRONOMY
    Michael Hoskin

THE HISTORY OF CHEMISTRY
William H. Brock
THE HISTORY OF CHILDHOOD
James Marten
THE HISTORY OF CINEMA
Geoffrey Nowell-Smith
THE HISTORY OF LIFE Michael Benton
THE HISTORY OF
MATHEMATICS Jacqueline Stedall
THE HISTORY OF MEDICINE
William Bynum
THE HISTORY OF PHYSICS
J. L. Heilbron
THE HISTORY OF TIME
Leofranc Holford-Strevens
HIV AND AIDS Alan Whiteside
HOBBES Richard Tuck
HOLLYWOOD Peter Decherney
THE HOLY ROMAN EMPIRE
Joachim Whaley
HOME Michael Allen Fox
HOMER Barbara Graziosi
HORMONES Martin Luck
HUMAN ANATOMY Leslie Klenerman
HUMAN EVOLUTION Bernard Wood
HUMAN RIGHTS Andrew Clapham
HUMANISM Stephen Law
HUME A. J. Ayer
HUMOUR Noël Carroll
THE ICE AGE Jamie Woodward
IDENTITY Florian Coulmas
IDEOLOGY Michael Freeden
THE IMMUNE SYSTEM
Paul Klenerman
INDIAN CINEMA Ashish Rajadhyaksha
INDIAN PHILOSOPHY Sue Hamilton
THE INDUSTRIAL REVOLUTION
Robert C. Allen
INFECTIOUS DISEASE Marta L. Wayne
and Benjamin M. Bolker
INFINITY Ian Stewart
INFORMATION Luciano Floridi
INNOVATION Mark Dodgson and
David Gann
INTELLECTUAL PROPERTY
Siva Vaidhyanathan
INTELLIGENCE Ian J. Deary
INTERNATIONAL LAW Vaughan Lowe
INTERNATIONAL MIGRATION
Khalid Koser

INTERNATIONAL RELATIONS
Paul Wilkinson
INTERNATIONAL SECURITY
Christopher S. Browning
IRAN Ali M. Ansari
ISLAM Malise Ruthven
ISLAMIC HISTORY Adam Silverstein
ISOTOPES Rob Ellam
ITALIAN LITERATURE
Peter Hainsworth and David Robey
JESUS Richard Bauckham
JEWISH HISTORY David N. Myers
JOURNALISM Ian Hargreaves
JUDAISM Norman Solomon
JUNG Anthony Stevens
KABBALAH Joseph Dan
KAFKA Ritchie Robertson
KANT Roger Scruton
KEYNES Robert Skidelsky
KIERKEGAARD Patrick Gardiner
KNOWLEDGE Jennifer Nagel
THE KORAN Michael Cook
LAKES Warwick F. Vincent
LANDSCAPE ARCHITECTURE
Ian H. Thompson
LANDSCAPES AND
GEOMORPHOLOGY
Andrew Goudie and Heather Viles
LANGUAGES Stephen R. Anderson
LATE ANTIQUITY Gillian Clark
LAW Raymond Wacks
THE LAWS OF THERMODYNAMICS
Peter Atkins
LEADERSHIP Keith Grint
LEARNING Mark Haselgrove
LEIBNIZ Maria Rosa Antognazza
LIBERALISM Michael Freeden
LIGHT Ian Walmsley
LINCOLN Allen C. Guelzo
LINGUISTICS Peter Matthews
LITERARY THEORY Jonathan Culler
LOCKE John Dunn
LOGIC Graham Priest
LOVE Ronald de Sousa
MACHIAVELLI Quentin Skinner
MADNESS Andrew Scull
MAGIC Owen Davies
MAGNA CARTA Nicholas Vincent
MAGNETISM Stephen Blundell
MALTHUS Donald Winch

MAMMALS T. S. Kemp
MANAGEMENT John Hendry
MAO Delia Davin
MARINE BIOLOGY Philip V. Mladenov
THE MARQUIS DE SADE John Phillips
MARTIN LUTHER Scott H. Hendrix
MARTYRDOM Jolyon Mitchell
MARX Peter Singer
MATERIALS Christopher Hall
MATHEMATICAL
  FINANCE Mark H. A. Davis
MATHEMATICS Timothy Gowers
MATTER Geoff Cottrell
THE MEANING OF LIFE
  Terry Eagleton
MEASUREMENT David Hand
MEDICAL ETHICS Michael Dunn and
  Tony Hope
MEDICAL LAW Charles Foster
MEDIEVAL BRITAIN John Gillingham
  and Ralph A. Griffiths
MEDIEVAL LITERATURE
  Elaine Treharne
MEDIEVAL PHILOSOPHY
  John Marenbon
MEMORY Jonathan K. Foster
METAPHYSICS Stephen Mumford
METHODISM William J. Abraham
THE MEXICAN REVOLUTION
  Alan Knight
MICHAEL FARADAY
  Frank A. J. L. James
MICROBIOLOGY Nicholas P. Money
MICROECONOMICS Avinash Dixit
MICROSCOPY Terence Allen
THE MIDDLE AGES Miri Rubin
MILITARY JUSTICE Eugene R. Fidell
MILITARY STRATEGY
  Antulio J. Echevarria II
MINERALS David Vaughan
MIRACLES Yujin Nagasawa
MODERN ARCHITECTURE
  Adam Sharr
MODERN ART David Cottington
MODERN CHINA Rana Mitter
MODERN DRAMA
  Kirsten E. Shepherd-Barr
MODERN FRANCE
  Vanessa R. Schwartz
MODERN INDIA Craig Jeffrey

MODERN IRELAND Senia Pašeta
MODERN ITALY Anna Cento Bull
MODERN JAPAN
  Christopher Goto-Jones
MODERN LATIN AMERICAN
  LITERATURE
  Roberto González Echevarría
MODERN WAR Richard English
MODERNISM Christopher Butler
MOLECULAR BIOLOGY Aysha Divan
  and Janice A. Royds
MOLECULES Philip Ball
MONASTICISM Stephen J. Davis
THE MONGOLS Morris Rossabi
MOONS David A. Rothery
MORMONISM Richard Lyman Bushman
MOUNTAINS Martin F. Price
MUHAMMAD Jonathan A. C. Brown
MULTICULTURALISM Ali Rattansi
MULTILINGUALISM John C. Maher
MUSIC Nicholas Cook
MYTH Robert A. Segal
NAPOLEON David Bell
THE NAPOLEONIC WARS
  Mike Rapport
NATIONALISM Steven Grosby
NATIVE AMERICAN LITERATURE
  Sean Teuton
NAVIGATION Jim Bennett
NELSON MANDELA Elleke Boehmer
NEOLIBERALISM Manfred Steger and
  Ravi Roy
NETWORKS Guido Caldarelli and
  Michele Catanzaro
THE NEW TESTAMENT
  Luke Timothy Johnson
THE NEW TESTAMENT AS
  LITERATURE Kyle Keefer
NEWTON Robert Iliffe
NIETZSCHE Michael Tanner
NINETEENTH-CENTURY
  BRITAIN Christopher Harvie and
  H. C. G. Matthew
THE NORMAN CONQUEST
  George Garnett
NORTH AMERICAN INDIANS
  Theda Perdue and Michael D. Green
NORTHERN IRELAND
  Marc Mulholland
NOTHING Frank Close

NUCLEAR PHYSICS Frank Close
NUCLEAR POWER Maxwell Irvine
NUCLEAR WEAPONS
    Joseph M. Siracusa
NUMBERS Peter M. Higgins
NUTRITION David A. Bender
OBJECTIVITY Stephen Gaukroger
OCEANS Dorrik Stow
THE OLD TESTAMENT
    Michael D. Coogan
THE ORCHESTRA D. Kern Holoman
ORGANIC CHEMISTRY
    Graham Patrick
ORGANIZATIONS Mary Jo Hatch
ORGANIZED CRIME
    Georgios A. Antonopoulos and
    Georgios Papanicolaou
PAGANISM Owen Davies
PAIN Rob Boddice
THE PALESTINIAN-ISRAELI
    CONFLICT Martin Bunton
PANDEMICS Christian W. McMillen
PARTICLE PHYSICS Frank Close
PAUL E. P. Sanders
PEACE Oliver P. Richmond
PENTECOSTALISM William K. Kay
PERCEPTION Brian Rogers
THE PERIODIC TABLE Eric R. Scerri
PHILOSOPHY Edward Craig
PHILOSOPHY IN THE ISLAMIC
    WORLD Peter Adamson
PHILOSOPHY OF LAW
    Raymond Wacks
PHILOSOPHY OF SCIENCE
    Samir Okasha
PHILOSOPHY OF RELIGION
    Tim Bayne
PHOTOGRAPHY Steve Edwards
PHYSICAL CHEMISTRY Peter Atkins
PHYSICS Sidney Perkowitz
PILGRIMAGE Ian Reader
PLAGUE Paul Slack
PLANETS David A. Rothery
PLANTS Timothy Walker
PLATE TECTONICS Peter Molnar
PLATO Julia Annas
POLITICAL PHILOSOPHY David Miller
POLITICS Kenneth Minogue
POPULISM Cas Mudde and
    Cristóbal Rovira Kaltwasser

POSTCOLONIALISM Robert Young
POSTMODERNISM Christopher Butler
POSTSTRUCTURALISM
    Catherine Belsey
POVERTY Philip N. Jefferson
PREHISTORY Chris Gosden
PRESOCRATIC PHILOSOPHY
    Catherine Osborne
PRIVACY Raymond Wacks
PROBABILITY John Haigh
PROGRESSIVISM Walter Nugent
PROJECTS Andrew Davies
PROTESTANTISM Mark A. Noll
PSYCHIATRY Tom Burns
PSYCHOANALYSIS Daniel Pick
PSYCHOLOGY Gillian Butler and
    Freda McManus
PSYCHOLOGY OF MUSIC
    Elizabeth Hellmuth Margulis
PSYCHOTHERAPY Tom Burns and
    Eva Burns-Lundgren
PUBLIC ADMINISTRATION
    Stella Z. Theodoulou and Ravi K. Roy
PUBLIC HEALTH Virginia Berridge
PURITANISM Francis J. Bremer
THE QUAKERS Pink Dandelion
QUANTUM THEORY
    John Polkinghorne
RACISM Ali Rattansi
RADIOACTIVITY Claudio Tuniz
RASTAFARI Ennis B. Edmonds
READING Belinda Jack
THE REAGAN REVOLUTION
    Gil Troy
REALITY Jan Westerhoff
THE REFORMATION Peter Marshall
RELATIVITY Russell Stannard
RELIGION IN AMERICA Timothy Beal
THE RENAISSANCE Jerry Brotton
RENAISSANCE ART
    Geraldine A. Johnson
REPTILES T. S. Kemp
REVOLUTIONS Jack A. Goldstone
RHETORIC Richard Toye
RISK Baruch Fischhoff and John Kadvany
RITUAL Barry Stephenson
RIVERS Nick Middleton
ROBOTICS Alan Winfield
ROCKS Jan Zalasiewicz
ROMAN BRITAIN Peter Salway

THE ROMAN EMPIRE
  Christopher Kelly
THE ROMAN REPUBLIC
  David M. Gwynn
ROMANTICISM Michael Ferber
ROUSSEAU Robert Wokler
RUSSELL A. C. Grayling
RUSSIAN HISTORY Geoffrey Hosking
RUSSIAN LITERATURE Catriona Kelly
THE RUSSIAN REVOLUTION
  S. A. Smith
THE SAINTS Simon Yarrow
SAVANNAS Peter A. Furley
SCHIZOPHRENIA Chris Frith and
  Eve Johnstone
SCHOPENHAUER
  Christopher Janaway
SCIENCE AND RELIGION
  Thomas Dixon
SCIENCE FICTION David Seed
THE SCIENTIFIC REVOLUTION
  Lawrence M. Principe
SCOTLAND Rab Houston
SEXUAL SELECTION Marlene Zuk and
  Leigh W. Simmons
SEXUALITY Véronique Mottier
SHAKESPEARE'S COMEDIES
  Bart van Es
SHAKESPEARE'S SONNETS AND
  POEMS Jonathan F. S. Post
SHAKESPEARE'S TRAGEDIES
  Stanley Wells
SIKHISM Eleanor Nesbitt
THE SILK ROAD James A. Millward
SLANG Jonathon Green
SLEEP Steven W. Lockley and
  Russell G. Foster
SOCIAL AND CULTURAL
  ANTHROPOLOGY
  John Monaghan and Peter Just
SOCIAL PSYCHOLOGY Richard J. Crisp
SOCIAL WORK Sally Holland and
  Jonathan Scourfield
SOCIALISM Michael Newman
SOCIOLINGUISTICS John Edwards
SOCIOLOGY Steve Bruce
SOCRATES C. C. W. Taylor
SOUND Mike Goldsmith
SOUTHEAST ASIA James R. Rush
THE SOVIET UNION Stephen Lovell

THE SPANISH CIVIL WAR
  Helen Graham
SPANISH LITERATURE Jo Labanyi
SPINOZA Roger Scruton
SPIRITUALITY Philip Sheldrake
SPORT Mike Cronin
STARS Andrew King
STATISTICS David J. Hand
STEM CELLS Jonathan Slack
STOICISM Brad Inwood
STRUCTURAL ENGINEERING
  David Blockley
STUART BRITAIN John Morrill
SUPERCONDUCTIVITY
  Stephen Blundell
SYMMETRY Ian Stewart
SYNAESTHESIA Julia Simner
SYNTHETIC BIOLOGY Jamie A. Davies
TAXATION Stephen Smith
TEETH Peter S. Ungar
TELESCOPES Geoff Cottrell
TERRORISM Charles Townshend
THEATRE Marvin Carlson
THEOLOGY David F. Ford
THINKING AND REASONING
  Jonathan St B. T. Evans
THOMAS AQUINAS Fergus Kerr
THOUGHT Tim Bayne
TIBETAN BUDDHISM
  Matthew T. Kapstein
TOCQUEVILLE Harvey C. Mansfield
TOLSTOY Liza Knapp
TRAGEDY Adrian Poole
TRANSLATION Matthew Reynolds
THE TREATY OF VERSAILLES
  Michael S. Neiberg
THE TROJAN WAR Eric H. Cline
TRUST Katherine Hawley
THE TUDORS John Guy
TWENTIETH-CENTURY
  BRITAIN Kenneth O. Morgan
TYPOGRAPHY Paul Luna
THE UNITED NATIONS
  Jussi M. Hanhimäki
UNIVERSITIES AND COLLEGES
  David Palfreyman and Paul Temple
THE U.S. CONGRESS
  Donald A. Ritchie
THE U.S. CONSTITUTION
  David J. Bodenhamer

THE U.S. SUPREME COURT
    Linda Greenhouse
UTILITARIANISM
    Katarzyna de Lazari-Radek
    and Peter Singer
UTOPIANISM Lyman Tower Sargent
VETERINARY SCIENCE James Yeates
THE VIKINGS Julian D. Richards
VIRUSES Dorothy H. Crawford
VOLTAIRE Nicholas Cronk
WAR AND TECHNOLOGY
    Alex Roland
WATER John Finney
WAVES Mike Goldsmith

WEATHER Storm Dunlop
THE WELFARE STATE David Garland
WILLIAM SHAKESPEARE
    Stanley Wells
WITCHCRAFT Malcolm Gaskill
WITTGENSTEIN A. C. Grayling
WORK Stephen Fineman
WORLD MUSIC Philip Bohlman
THE WORLD TRADE
    ORGANIZATION Amrita Narlikar
WORLD WAR II Gerhard L. Weinberg
WRITING AND SCRIPT
    Andrew Robinson
ZIONISM Michael Stanislawski

Available soon:

PSYCHOPATHY Essi Viding
NAZI GERMANY Jane Caplan
POETRY Bernard O'Donoghue

ENERGY SYSTEMS
    Nick Jenkins
DYNASTY JEROEN DUINDAM

For more information visit our website

www.oup.com/vsi/

Julia Simner

SYNAESTHESIA

A Very Short Introduction

OXFORD
UNIVERSITY PRESS

OXFORD

UNIVERSITY PRESS

Great Clarendon Street, Oxford, OX2 6DP,
United Kingdom

Oxford University Press is a department of the University of Oxford.
It furthers the University's objective of excellence in research, scholarship,
and education by publishing worldwide. Oxford is a registered trade mark of
Oxford University Press in the UK and in certain other countries

First edition published in 2019

Impression: 2

Published in the United States of America by Oxford University Press
198 Madison Avenue, New York, NY 10016, United States of America

British Library Cataloguing in Publication Data
Data available

Library of Congress Control Number: 2019936329

ISBN 978-0-19-874921-9

Printed in Great Britain by
Ashford Colour Press Ltd, Gosport, Hampshire

To Bally, for the marvellous surprise.

Contents

Preface and acknowledgements xvii

List of illustrations xix

1 What is synaesthesia? 1

2 Synaesthesia in the brain 20

3 Synaesthesia and the arts 43

4 Is synaesthesia a 'gift' or a 'condition'? 62

5 Where does synaesthesia come from? The role of genetics and learning 83

6 The question of synaesthesia 105

Further reading and references 117

Index 125

Preface and acknowledgements

As a 6-year-old boy, James Wannerton would sometimes wonder why he tasted blackcurrants when he heard his sister's name. Or why the name of the London Underground station at Piccadilly Circus flooded his mouth with the taste of chewy peanut chocolate. As an adult James one day heard a word that would change his life. He learned about *synaesthesia*, contacted a scientist, took part in research, and finally got the answers he was looking for. James tasted words because the taste centres in his brain were different to the average person. He went on to be one of the founding members of the UK Synaesthesia Association, a collaboration between synaesthetes, scientists, and artists which seeks to further the study of synaesthesia and to widen public understanding. Today James Wannerton is the President of the UK Synaesthesia Association and I am a professor of neuropsychology who serves as its Science Officer. This book is the story of this extraordinary condition: an explanation of what synaesthesia is, how it manifests itself, what causes it, how it feels, how it links to creativity and the arts, and what it can tell us about every human's perceptions of reality. My hope in writing this book is that future 6-year-old boys (or girls!) needn't wonder for too long, if they have a rare and special mixing of the senses.

I first heard the word 'synaesthesia' over twenty years ago and I have since had the pleasure and interest of studying thousands of cases—all synaesthetes, all unique—who have kindly taken time to share their experiences with me. I have responded to countless emails, written scores of science papers, answered hundreds of questions from synaesthetes, from their parents, from the media, from university students, from school children, from colleagues, and of course from my own friends and family. In writing this book, I owe special thanks to all the synaesthetes who have shared their stories with me, and especially to those who have taken time out of their busy lives to take part in my psychology studies. I apologize to them for sweeping statements in this book if they do not seem to ring true for every synaesthete reader. I have described what current science can tell us about synaesthetes in general, but acknowledge that synaesthetes are, of course, also individuals.

Among the synaesthetes I have met, I am especially grateful to James Wannerton, Sean Day, Carol Steen, and Patricia Lynne Duffy who have served as, variously, founders or presidents of the UK and US Synaesthesia Associations—as well as to the teams who support them and the numerous synaesthesia associations around the world. Their generosity of time and their determination to spread the word about synaesthesia have provided a potential platform of expression to over 300 million synaesthetes worldwide. I am grateful too for the support from Oxford University Press in writing this book. And I would like to thank my students and lab-team; they provide an inspiring intellectual environment to work in and teach me something new every day. Along with them I'd like to thank my collaborator Jamie Ward who has shown me, with his great intellectual generosity over the last twenty years, how the very best scientists should work. Many of the advances in this field have been guided by his insights. Finally I am most grateful to Iain, Tommy, Indy, Alex, Jean, Edwin, Jo, and Vickie. Some of these have fascinated me with their orange Wednesdays, golden Fridays, and tweed-textured Tuesdays, but mostly they have asked me questions and given me their support on the home front. So this book is for my family, and for synaesthetes everywhere.

List of illustrations

1 Synaesthetic shapes and textures triggered by four sounds **7**

Reproduced with permission from Layden, TB., et al. Comparing the Shape of Sounds: An artistic Investigation. *Proceeding of the V International Conference on Synesthesia, Science and Art*. Alcalá la Real, 16–19th May 2015. Copyright © 2015, The Authors.

2 Examples of sequence-space synaesthesia **10**

Reproduced with permission from Simner J., et al. A foundation for savantism? Visuo-spatial synaesthetes present with cognitive benefits. *Cortex*, 45(10): 1246–1260. Copyright © 2009 Elsevier Srl. All rights reserved. https://doi.org/10.1016/j.cortex.2009.07.007. Courtesy of JSTOR. Available at: https://archive.org/details/jstor-1411774.

3 The human brain's four lobes: temporal, frontal, parietal, and occipital **22**

4 PET scanner **24**

schoolphysics.co.uk.

5 fMRI brain scans of a synaesthete and a non-synaesthete **29**

Reproduced with permission from Hubbard, EM., et al. Individual Differences among Grapheme-Color Synesthetes: Brain-Behavior Correlations. *Neuron*, 45(6): 975–985 © 2015, Cell Press. Copyright © 2005 Elsevier Inc. All rights reserved. https://doi.org/10.1016/j.neuron.2005.02.008.

6 A neuron **35**

ALFRED PASIEKA / Science Photo Library RF / age fotostock.

7 Diagnostic test for lexical-gustatory synaesthesia **53**

8 *Dark Glistening* **57**

Timothy B Layden, 2010. Oil on Canvas, 100x100 cm. http://theshapeofsounds.com.

9 Still frames from an animation showing the shapes of sounds **60**

Reproduced with permission from Ward, J., et al. The Aesthetic Appeal of Auditory-Visual Synaesthetic Perceptions in People without Synaesthesia. *Perception*, 37(8): 1285–1296. Copyright © 2008, © SAGE Publications. https://doi.org/10.1068/p5815.

10 Experimental set-up to study mirror-touch synaesthesia **75**

Reproduced with permission from Medina, J., and DePasquale, C. Influence of the body schema on mirror-touch synaesthesia. *Cortex*, 88: 53–65. Copyright © 2016 Elsevier Ltd. All rights reserved. https://doi.org/10.1016/j.cortex.2016.12.013.

11 *Tastes of London* 1964–2013 **77**

James Wannerton.

12 Daniel Tammet's synaesthetic number landscape for π **82**

Pi Landscape by Daniel Tammet. http://danieltammet.net/.

13 A representation of the prototypical synaesthetic colour(s) for letters **85**

14 Experimental set-up to study cross-modal correspondence between touch and vision **93**

15 The 3D structure of DNA **96**

iStock.com / lvcandy.

Chapter 1
What is synaesthesia?

James Wannerton was born on 18 February 1959 in Manchester, England. He has grown up to become the President of the UK Synaesthesia Association, an organization founded in 1989 to support and inform people with synaesthesia, and he still holds that role at the time of my writing this book. Because James was born with synaesthesia he is an unusual member of the population—but in many ways, James is a fairly typical person who has had a fairly typical life. As a child he loved to watch TV and play soccer like most English boys. His first job out of school was as a computer operator back in the days when a computer was the size of a room, but he has worked in numerous jobs throughout his adult life: from graphic designer to pub owner. And James has remained a perfectly ordinary individual in almost every way—except that for as long as he can remember, James has experienced phantom tastes in his mouth. These tastes are triggered every time James hears words. Indeed tastes are so inherently associated with words that James tastes every word he reads, speaks, hears, or even thinks about. Each word in English floods his mouth with a different flavour sensation—as do some sounds, and many words in languages he does not even speak. When James hears the word 'audience' for example, his mouth is flooded with the taste of peas. The name 'Phillip' fills his mouth with bitter oranges. And the word 'society' tastes of onions. These flavours are triggered by unusual features within James' brain, but the tastes are as true, rounded, and 'real' as any flavours of food you might put in your mouth—except of course there's nothing in James's mouth when he tastes them. The tastes are triggered by the sounds of words because James has a form of synaesthesia.

Synaesthesia (whose American spelling is 'synesthesia') is often described as a rare neurological condition that gives rise to a type of 'merging of the senses'. For those who experience it—people called *synaesthetes*—one sense appears to merge or cross with another. Synaesthesia is a multi-variant condition meaning it has many different ways of presenting itself, and this means there are many different types of synaesthete. Some synaesthetes, like James, taste words (and this is called *lexical-gustatory synaesthesia*). Others see colours when they hear sounds (*sound-colour synaesthesia*). Some see colours in response to the tastes of food they eat, or from their sense of touch when they feel different textures against their fingertips (*flavour-colour* and *touch-colour synaesthesia*, respectively). And yet others hear sounds when they see silent moving objects (*visual-auditory synaesthesia*). In fact, different synaesthetes experience many different types of sensation and the number of different types of synaesthesias that have been counted lies somewhere between one and two hundred at least—although there may be many more. But in our last screening for 128 different types, the number of people with synaesthesia amounted to just 4.4 per cent of the population. This rare condition appears to affect men and women in equal numbers, although it was once thought to be an especially female trait. However, recent studies show that female synaesthetes are simply more likely to *come forward* to report their unusual experiences. Female synaesthetes therefore appear more often than men as volunteers in research studies, but this difference disappears when we screen for synaesthesia in the general population.

Because synaesthesia is rare, the majority of the people reading this page will be doing so with a sense of unfamiliarity and perhaps even scepticism. If we imagine the traditional five senses of sight, hearing, taste, touch, and smell, most people tend to experience them as separate entities: noise makes a sound but it doesn't have a taste! Colour is something that can be seen but not heard! This clean segregation of the world is what gives most people their solid sense of reality. And this reality feels fixed and permanent: the colour red looks red, salt taste salty, shrill noises sound shrill—and we have the unerring impression that anybody else standing in our shoes would experience the world in exactly the same way. But our perception of the world is filtered through the individuality of our brain. And because some brains differ in subtle ways, some people experience the world as a qualitatively different place. And synaesthesia is a case in point. In the chapters that follow we will see that the brains of synaesthetes have a type of 'rerouting' of information: signals from the eyes are reaching the hearing centres of the brain; signals from the ears are reaching colour centres; and so on. And because of this, synaesthesia can provide intriguing information about how the mind interprets reality, by relying not only on external information from the outside world, but an internal reorganization of that information as it enters the brain. To understand this we will have to realize that the human brain is *never* a passive device merely observing the world, but that *every* human brain is an active manipulator of what we see around us, constantly organizing the incoming signals in certain ways. Synaesthesia simply arises when that organization is different. So throughout this book I shall describe many types of synaesthesia and explain exactly why and how synaesthesia occurs, and how it conjures up a different sensory reality for the people who experience it.

Synaesthesia—not one condition but many

Synaesthesia has always been a challenge to define, most immediately because it refers to a large number of different experiences. Synaesthetes can feel unusual colours, tastes, smells, shapes, textures, and a number of other sensory experiences, not

3

to mention abstract sensations involving emotions and thoughts (more on this below). Moreover, these synaesthetic experiences can be triggered by a range of activities, including reading, eating, counting, moving, swimming, speaking, listening to music, or even just sitting and thinking quietly. But at its core, synaesthesia is the automatic linking of sensations that the average person does not usually experience together. It is when one quality of experience is accompanied by an involuntary unrelated secondary experience (e.g. hearing sounds gives rise to seeing colours). Above we described this as a 'merging of the senses' but this commonly-used definition is inaccurate in a number of ways. First, the sensations do not merge—they simply co-occur. So when I speak to James Wannerton, he clearly hears the words I pronounce as sounds in the normal way, but he also experiences tastes in his mouth. The tastes are triggered by my words but taste and sound do not blur—they simply co-exist. So it is not so much a 'merging of the senses' as a 'pairing of the senses', with one sense triggering another, and importantly, in a way that is rare in the population and linked to brain differences. Another common feature of synaesthesia is that the sensations experienced by any given synaesthete tend to remain consistent over time. So for James Wannerton, the word 'society' always triggers the same taste of onions; the word 'audience' always triggers the same taste of peas; and the word 'Phillip' always tastes of bitter oranges. Each word and taste remain firmly locked together, and this *consistency over time* is assumed to be pervasive across all synaesthesias. Indeed it is such an important trait that we will return to it many times in this book.

Another archetypal example of synaesthesia is sound-colour synaesthesia. I should point out that here and throughout this book I am following the widely held convention of naming a synaesthesia by placing the trigger before the synaesthetic sensation. So sound-colour synaesthesia is triggered by sound and causes unusual sensations of colour. The trigger is often called the *inducer* of synaesthesia, and the unusual associated sensation experienced as a result is called the *concurrent*. For sound-colour synaesthetes then, hearing sounds induces the concurrent of colour. Sound-colour synaesthesia perfectly fits the definition of synaesthesia I have given above because there is a bringing together of two senses (hearing and vision), the experience is rare (only 0.2 per cent of the population experience colours from sounds), and those who experience it have neurological differences in their brains compared to the average person, which we will explore later. This variant is sometimes known as *music-colour synaesthesia* because it is often triggered by listening to music. But what are these colours like exactly? Descriptions given by music-colour synaesthetes suggest they can form specific shapes and patterns, and they can move around in the visual field, waxing and waning with changes in the music that triggers them.

In explaining the quality of synaesthetic colours I am reminded of a story told to me at a conference dinner by Julian Asher, a sound-colour synaesthete who is also a synaesthesia scientist. As a geneticist, he pioneered the first genetics research into synaesthesia in 2009, and he himself experiences synaesthetic colours in response to the different timbres of musical instruments. So for Julian Asher, piano music is a deep purple colour, cellos make music that is the colour of golden honey, and violins are the burgundy colour of red wine. These colours are so tangibly real for Julian that as a child he assumed they were part of the general experiences of everyone. When Julian's parents took him to the symphony as a young boy, he always supposed that the house-lights dimmed before the performance began so the audience could see the colours better. ('Why else would they do it?' he said.) This assumption was natural to Julian because his synaesthetic colours have a 'veridical' quality—they are real to Julian Asher and to many other synaesthetes who experience them. And yet just as there is more than one type of synaesthesia, there is also more than one type of synaesthete—even among those experiencing the same pairings (e.g. sound and colour). So some synaesthetes see their unusual colours as if these were real entities in the outside world, while others see them as mental images in their mind's eye. Still other synaesthetes have no sense of seeing or imaging at all—they simply have a strong sense of knowing what the colours *must be*. These differences in how the colour is experienced have been captured by psychologist Mike Dixon and his colleagues with their distinction between *projector* and *associator* synaesthetes: projectors see colours like external objects somewhere out in space, while associators have colours that are just 'known' or seen in the mind's eye. We shall see in Chapter 2 that this quality can even be read off brain scans because differences in the way synaesthetes experience their colours are matched by differences in the connections within their brains. And whether the colours are internal or external, the differences do not stop here. Some describe their synaesthesia as being on an 'external screen', others as projected onto some object in the outside world, like a written word. Synaesthetic users of sign language have reported colours projected onto the fingertips when signing letters. And a student of mine from a decade ago described how her synaesthetic colours (this time produced by the pain of a headache) appeared to project from her head in the shape of a cone. If she thought hard about the shape she could even soften the headache.

Colours themselves appear to be by far the most common type of synaesthetic sensation overall in terms of reported cases (although colours might simply be the easiest sensations for synaesthetes to describe, which would make them appear more common than they actually are). But colour is just one of the sensations experienced by synaesthetes. In fact, 'sound-colour synaesthesia' is something of a misnomer because its synaesthetic colours tend to also be accompanied by other sensations such as moving shapes and textures. Examples of these shapes can be seen in Figure 1, drawn by sound-colour synaesthete Christine Söffing to show her synaesthetic shapes triggered by four different sounds ((1) an oscillating bass sound moving from loudly low pitch to quietly high pitch; (2) a static-filled electronic sound growing louder then quieter; (3) a metallic ringing with resonant echoes;

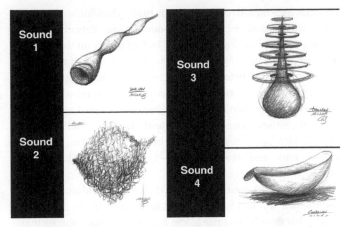

1. Images drawn by artist Christine Söffing to capture her synaesthetic shapes and textures triggered by four sounds.

and (4) rhythmic electronic record scratches). As an artist, Söffing has the observational skills and dexterity to represent her synaesthetic experiences using different artistic media. Her images also attempt to capture the movement and morphing of shapes, which for her change over time or in response to the dynamic qualities of the sound.

Aside from colour and shape, synaesthetes might also experience synaesthetic sounds triggered by looking at silent moving objects. These moving objects can sometimes be heard to 'whoosh' in the minds of synaesthetes, or make other sounds like whirring or buzzing. Alternatively, synaesthetes might experience sensations such as touch. Touch was the particular experience in a well-known case of synaesthesia captured in the book *The Man Who Tasted Shapes* written by neurologist Richard Cytowic. This book details a case that has entered synaesthesia folk-lore not only because it was so comprehensively described by the author, but because Richard Cytowic was interested in synaesthesia at a time when nobody else was looking at synaesthesia at all. The true events in his book date back to one evening in 1980, when Richard Cytowic was invited to dinner by his neighbour Michael Watson. During dinner, Michael apologized for the lack of points on the chicken. To most people this might be an unusual comment, but worthy only of a puzzled pause before the conversation moved on again. But for Richard Cytowic, trained as a neurologist, it sparked a distant memory of a condition he had once heard about called 'synaesthesia' where the senses appear to cross. Cytowic asked Michael Watson about his feelings of touch triggered by flavours and then went on to study him—and his synaesthesia—for the next three decades.

Michael Watson's synaesthesia was described over dinner because for Michael, flavours have shapes. The intensity of the flavour of food in his mouth gives rise to the feeling of abstract shapes that rub against his face, sweep down his arm, and come to rest in his palms. Michael can feel in his hands the synaesthetic shape of the food, its synaesthetic weight, its synaesthetic texture. And he knew exactly what a good-tasting chicken should be like—it should be pointed, but his chicken had come out all round. And by voicing his disappointment, Michael Watson sparked a field of science. Richard Cytowic's detailed descriptions and careful experiments went on to form the basis for a number of books and science articles. And partly as a result of these efforts, over 500 academic articles have since been written about the psychology, neuroscience, prevalence, development, genetics, aesthetics, and history of synaesthesia. The answers that scientists and other scholars have been able to generate about this fascinating phenomenon will fill the pages of this book.

Michael Watson's geometric tastes and Julian Asher's coloured music are both archetypal synaesthesias, each bringing together two of the five senses: taste-touch and sound-sight respectively. These manifestations are therefore aptly captured by our characterization of synaesthesia as a 'pairing of the senses'. But interestingly, other kinds of synaesthesia do not fit this definition in any easy way. Describing synaesthesia as a 'pairing of the senses' belies the fact that a large number of synaesthesias are triggered by things that are not from the five senses at all. Consider for example *sequence-space synaesthesia*. This takes the first half of its name from the fact that the synaesthesia is triggered by ordered sequences in language, such as letters (ordered ABC...), numbers (ordered 123...), months of the year (ordered January, February, March...) or other sequences like days of the week and so on. These sequences are particularly strong triggers of synaesthesia and in sequence-space synaesthesia they cause a synaesthetic concurrent that is spatial in nature. So synaesthetes with sequence-space synaesthesia have the impression that letters, number, months, etc., are laid out in space in particular spatial patterns (sometimes called 'visuo-spatial forms'). I have given several examples in Figure 2(a). These examples were taken from a study I conducted with colleagues Neil Mayo and Mary-Jane Spiller in 2009 about a group of sequence-space synaesthetes whose spatial forms happen to be triggered by sequences of time in particular (e.g. days, months, years).

One remarkable thing about sequence-space synaesthesia—and indeed about synaesthesia in general—is that the descriptions given by synaesthetes are similar from country to country, continent to continent, and indeed from century to century. This particular variant of synaesthesia was first described in the 19th century, and examples of sequence-space patterns from this earlier era can be found in Figure 2(b). These examples were taken from a report written by researcher D. E. Phillips in 1897 and yet another early account comes from Sir Francis Galton in 1880. Galton was a polymath and cousin of Charles Darwin, who wrote over 300 books and science papers during his lifetime on topics as varied as meteorology (he constructed the first weather map) to criminology (he pioneered a fingerprinting technique still used today). But Galton always had a fascination for the human mind, and in 1880 he focussed on sequence-space synaesthesia, especially as triggered by numbers. In his reports he described

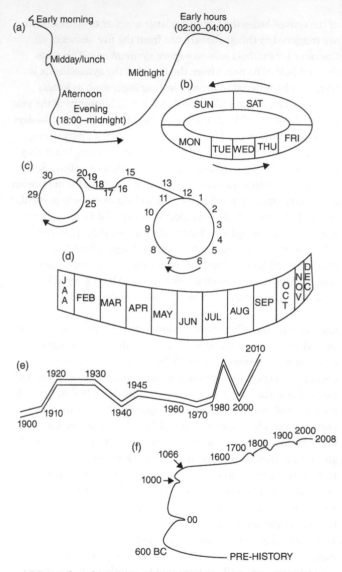

2. (a) Examples of sequence-space synaesthesia: clockwise from top left showing hours within a day, days within a week, days within a month, months within a year, years within a century, and centuries within millennia.

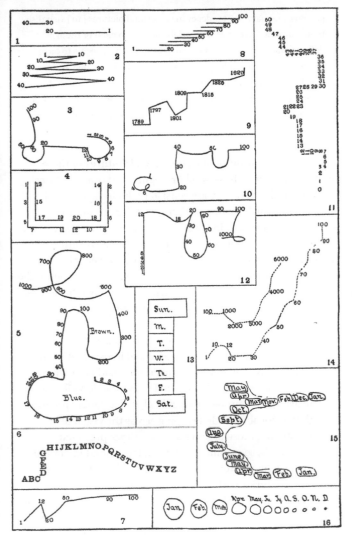

2. (b) examples of sequence-space synaesthesia from 19th-century synaesthetes showing numbers, letters, days within a week, months within a year, and years within centuries.

persons who have the tendency to use mental pictures [to] visualise their numerals ... but also invariably assign to each of them a definite place in their mental field of view, where it seems to have a home. Thus 6 may always lie low down to the left, 7 may be found a little higher and more to the front, and so on. It follows that whenever these persons think of a series of numbers, as 1, 2, 3, 4, 5 &c., they always appear to the mind's eye as ranged in a definite pattern or 'form'.

In his reports, Galton pointed out several features of these number forms, which we would recognize today as qualities of synaesthesia: that they are consistent, lifelong, unusual experiences, which bring together two different qualities (sequences and space) in a way not experienced by the average person. And like other synaesthesias they are also automatic, in that synaesthetes do not have to consciously invent them or make any effort to conjure them up. They just appear when the synaesthete is thinking about sequences, and it will have been that way ever since the synaesthete was young.

Figures 2(a) and 2(b) show that the mental shapes of sequence-space synaesthetes are varied and idiosyncratic but all share a quality in common. Sequences are laid out in fixed patterns, with curves, bends, and angles, as time flows forwards and backwards, as numbers rise and fall, and as letters progress through the alphabet while sweeping across the visual field. For synaesthetes, these patterns are sometimes projected in front of the body, sometimes even wrapping around it. For one synaesthete, who is referred to in the science literature by his initials IB, centuries within the last millennium rise up in columns in front of his body. If IB reaches out his left hand at hip height he can touch the location of the year 1700, which rests about a foot in front of his body and around 3 feet off the ground. Raising his hand to touch his nose with his forefinger traces the path of the 1700s, all the way up to 1799 where the column breaks as the century ends. The year 1800 starts again way down in front of him, back again at hip height just to the right of the century that came before. And so it goes on: IB's centuries rise up to meet him, in tilted columns stacked next to each other from left to right in the space in front of his body. But something unusual happened to IB at the start of the 21st century. He noticed one day that, curiously, the year 2000 had not gone back to base at hip height but instead was carrying on at the top of the column immediately above 1999. A few years later he realized the 21st century was progressing steadfastly over his right shoulder. By 2013 he could barely see the top of the column without turning his head. In 2019 the years have curved very slightly out of sight behind him. 'Where are they going next?' I asked. 'I don't know' he said ... 'I don't make the rules'.

What is particularly important for our purposes here is to note that this synaesthesia is triggered by thinking about sequences, and this does not constitute a sensory act. In other words the trigger for this synaesthesia does not involve the five senses of hearing, seeing, tasting, smelling, or touching but is what psychologists would refer to as an act of *cognition*. Clearly then, our definition of synaesthesia as a 'pairing of the senses' fails in this case because what has triggered this synaesthesia is not a sense at all. So what are the implications for our definition of synaesthesia? One solution is to say that this type of experience is not synaesthesia at all—precisely because there are no *senses* paired together and because we might wish to keep the definition in some way 'pure'. But a pure definition is of limited use if it does not capture the full spectrum of manifestations. And continuing to insist on a definition that involves the senses would also exclude some of the most widely-accepted synaesthesias by far. *Grapheme-colour synaesthesia* affects 1 to 2 per cent of the population and causes letters and numbers (i.e. graphemes) to be imbued with colours. So the letter A might trigger the colour red, or the number 3 might trigger blue. This is the best understood and best described synaesthesia by far, and its synaesthetic status has never once been in doubt. But it too defies the definition of a 'pairing of senses' because its trigger is the abstract concept of a letter or number. We can demonstrate this easily by altering the sensory qualities of the trigger and showing that the synaesthesia remains largely the same. So the letter A would be the same synaesthetic colour whether it is printed in UPPERCASE or lowercase and irrespective of font (a or a), all of which change the letter's visual qualities. And the letter A would stay the same colour whether pronounced '*a as-in-ca*t' or '*a as-in-a*rch' all of which change the letter's auditory qualities. So sensory qualities do not seem to matter suggesting that grapheme-colour synaesthesia, too, is something other than a pairing of the *senses*. (By the way, if you are reading this and do have very different synaesthetic colours for 'A' depending on how it is pronounced, then you are not a grapheme-colour synaesthete but a *phoneme-colour synaesthete*—a different form entirely.)

So sequence-space synaesthesia is not a one-off oddity in resisting the definition of a 'pairing of senses'; many other types of synaesthesias do the same. Another example is *sequence-personality synaesthesia*. As the name suggests, this too is triggered by ordered linguistic sequences although this time, the synaesthetic concurrent is a personality or gender. So for sequence-personality synaesthetes, numbers (or letters, or months, etc.) are a complex cast of characters. They have their own personalities, their own ages, genders, interests, and dispositions. For the synaesthete known as AP for example, who was kind enough to take part in my study in 2006, the number 1 is male and 'a good guy'; synaesthete AP has the unquestionable impression that he is a responsible man who acts like a father figure to the other numbers, being very nice but rather tired. Number 7 is also a man but weak and submissive and rather unconfident; while number 5 is a mother figure who works hard around the house but occasionally does funny things by accident. This soap opera of characters continues into her letters: *E* and *f* are roguish young men but although *e* is charming, *f* is sinister. The letter *i* is a young boy

14

fussed over by *h* and *g*. But all he really wants is to be independent and to get on in life. And the months of the year, too, run through a cast of characters, from *January* (the sensible one) to *December* (the boss).

Accounts of sequence-personality synaesthesia (also known as *ordinal linguistic personification* or *OLP*) date back over a hundred years. Perhaps the most detailed historical report was written in 1893 by a Swiss neuroscientist called Théodore Flournoy. A decade ago, my colleague Edward Hubbard and I took on the challenge of translating Flournoy's writings from their original French, and what we found was a remarkably modern account, with all the same markers we might recognize in the recent cases I had come across myself. Here is our translation of how Flournoy described an individual he interviewed named 'Madame L'. We know very little about who she was except that she was well-educated, 46 years of age, in good health, and a sequence-personality synaesthete.

Madame L. has always personified numbers, to the point where she could easily write a novel about some of them. She says 1, 2, 3 are children without fixed personalities; they play together. Number 4 is a good peaceful woman, absorbed by down-to-earth occupations and who takes pleasure in them. 5 is a young man, ordinary and common in his tastes and appearance....6 is a young man of 16 or 17 years of age, very well brought up, polite, gentle, agreeable in appearance, and with upstanding tastes; average intelligence; orphan. 7 is a bad sort, although brought up well; spiritual, extravagant... 8 is a dignified lady, who acts appropriately, and who is linked with 7 and has much influence on him. She is the wife of 9. 9 is the husband of Madame 8. He is self-centred, maniacal, selfish, thinks only about himself, is grumpy, endlessly reproaching his wife for one thing or another; telling her, for example, that he would have been better to have married a 9, since between them they would have made 18–as opposed to only 17 with her... Number 10, and the other remaining numerals, have no personifications.

What we find in all these cases are in-depth descriptions, and this is another key feature of synaesthesia. Throughout this book we will see that synaesthetic experiences are clear and detailed in the minds of synaesthetes. The synaesthetic personalities described by Madame L are so detailed and so real that we might even start to feel sorry for poor old number 8, with her unhappy marriage to 9 and mysterious links to the dubious number 7. Of course all people have some ability to project personalities onto inanimate objects: we might feel that a constantly crashing computer is holding a grudge, or that a newly christened boat is likely to be given a female name. But in Chapter 2 we will see that the extreme projections of sequence-personality synaesthesia appear to lie in differences in connections within the corpus callosum—an area of the brain linking left and right hemispheres which differs subtly in the brains of such synaesthetes.

But if there is no *sensory* merging in sequence-personality synaesthesia (both inducer and concurrent are non-sensory) should this be considered a synaesthesia at all? There are reasons to believe it should, although the field is divided here. In my own view, sequence-personality holds the very essence of synaesthesia by uniting two qualities that the average person does not experience together (sequences and personalities) giving lifelong, automatic associations, which are highly detailed, intensely experienced, and triggered by what we might consider the synaesthetic trigger par excellence (ordered sequences). Like other synaesthesias, it is stable over time, and (as we will see in Chapter 2) tied to differences in the structural connectivity of the brain. To me it seems to be everything that characterizes synaesthesia as we understand it today. Most importantly sequence-personality synaesthesia is especially experienced by those who happen to have other forms of synaesthesia too. This is important because in our chapter on genetics we will see that multiple forms of synaesthesia tend to cluster within individuals. Everything about this experience is resonant of what synaesthesia is considered to be, so let us take it as such for now—although it is important to note that some scientists may not agree.

We end this chapter without controversy by describing a final example of synaesthesia that does indeed cross the senses. Sean Day is a scientist who has a number of synaesthesias including colours triggered by the smell and taste of food in his mouth. When Sean Day eats raw spinach he sees deep purple. When he eats beef the colour is dark blue. Chicken is cyan, and almonds are bright orange. Suffice it to say that these colours are not reflective of the foods themselves: brown sauce triggers a grey colour, raspberries trigger orange, oranges trigger a blue colour, and so on. His synaesthetic colours swirl up in front of him at eye-level, and many are close enough that he can immerse his hands into them. Perhaps most remarkably, their quality is real enough to Sean Day that his can swirl his fingers around in them until the colours start to move and swirl themselves. And the quality of colour is so robust that Sean often cannot see through them until they start to dissipate of their own accord—about four or five seconds after they have first appeared.

I chose this case as our final example because it shows how synaesthesia can have an effect on lives, in both subtle and important ways. Synaesthesia influences Sean Day's buying behaviours, for example. He tends to buy cheese in blue containers, regardless of whether he likes the type of cheese on offer. He will gravitate towards coffee in dark green packaging and he will buy chicken with labels that are blue. These behavioural choices are dictated by his synaesthesia because matching real-world colours with synaesthetic ones makes things 'feel right'. And synaesthesia affects Sean Day in other ways too. When he drives, particularly strong smells cause him to pull over because he cannot easily see through the colours they have triggered. Similarly, James Wannerton finds driving difficult, because words on road signs can flood his mouth with strong flavours—which he has to try to ignore when concentrating on the road. James also avoids busy places because the hubbub of noise can overwhelm his taste buds. (We once had lunch together by the side of the Niagara Falls and I was mindful to keep my dinner-table chit-chat to a minimum—who knows what types of flavours I'd be imposing in his mouth by talking as he was eating. But as it turns out, I needn't have bothered—all the while I was quiet, he was tasting porridge from the sound of the waterfalls crashing down beside us.)

And synaesthesia can influence lives in other ways. Sean Day also experiences coloured music and sought out instruments from an early age for the qualities of their synaesthetic colours. He later became an accomplished musician. Conversely, James Wannerton was forced to give up a nascent career as a pub owner because the constant swirl of tastes, smells, and sounds—both real and synaesthetic in his noisy pub—became overwhelming. It also affected his social life. James finds himself avoiding people whose names taste particularly bad (his friend Derek tasted of ear-wax), and if he cannot avoid it he tries to compensate in other ways. So although most of my friends and colleagues use the short form of my name, Jools, it is James alone who calls me Julia; it has a far better taste of orange fruit sweets, compared to the lumpy wallpaper-paste of Jools. And so it goes on. The pleasing or displeasing colours, flavours, shapes, and other sensations which are part of the ever-present nature of synaesthesia have formed behaviours, broken friendships, stimulated musical talents, influenced careers, and even named babies. They have had all manner of impact on the lives of synaesthetes, because synaesthetes are as sensitive to nice or nasty sensations as anyone else—although in the case of synaesthesia, these sensations are internally generated.

Synaesthesia—what's in a name?

We have seen in this chapter that synaesthesia can manifest in many different ways, and this poses a challenge for scientists in setting out a definition. The name synaesthesia itself comes from two Greek words: σύν (syn, meaning 'together') and αἴσθησις (aisthēsis, meaning 'sensation') but we have seen that inducers and concurrents can be all manner of sensations, or even intangible concepts of personality, meaning, space, and time. Whether all these experiences should be considered as forms of synaesthesia I will leave the reader to decide, but for now we will continue with this widely held framework throughout the book. And our focus throughout will be largely what is known as *developmental* or *congenital synaesthesia*; cases where synaesthesia emerges spontaneously in early childhood, the person apparently predisposed in some way from birth. Rarer instances have been reported of *acquired synaesthesia*, which is the emergence of synaesthesia in later life triggered by some life event such as the onset of disease—or as we will see in Chapter 2, even drug use.

If most readers of this book are non-synaesthetes, the accounts I have given here might seem unusual. But as writer Patricia Lynn Duffy observed, 'anyone expecting that such...words would come from the mind of a quirky eccentric would be very much on the wrong track. [Synaesthetes are often] serious, straightforward, self-assured, and also searching'. This has also been my own observation, too, of many of the synaesthetes I have met over the last two decades. In the following chapters we will look at what causes synaesthesia in terms of neural biology, and we will find out what questions can be answered by looking directly into brains of synaesthetes.

Chapter 2
Synaesthesia in the brain

Advances in brain imaging have revolutionized the study of synaesthesia and have enormous potential in educating us about the aetiology of this unusual condition. Brain imaging has also changed the way synaesthesia is viewed by both scientists and the population at large, and I have seen for myself the impact of each new neuroscientific discovery on the way synaesthesia has risen in public awareness. Brain scans provide clear and irrefutable evidence of how synaesthetic sensations are grounded in the brain, in a way that can be easily understood and not easily dismissed. When I first made synaesthesia the focus of my academic career almost two decades ago I would spend most of my talks at science conferences simply trying to demonstrate that synaesthesia was real. But with the advent of brain scanning I no longer had to work hard around the 'genuineness' issue—I could start with one slide showing the scan of a synaesthete's brain and then move on to the rest of my talk. So something that audiences once grappled with as an existential challenge now has a robust and accepted neuroscientific basis with known characteristics that can be widely understood, not only by scientists but also the general public. And so this is the topic we turn to now: brain imaging.

Sensations in the brain

In Chapter 1, I said that to understand synaesthesia we must understand that colours, sounds, tastes, and other sensations that appear to come from the outside world are actually generated in our own brains. To understand this, imagine you need to post a letter. You go out onto the street to look for a post-box, which in the UK will be bright red. You spot the familiar red colour of the post-box and head towards it. You probably think the reason you are seeing the colour red is because the colour exists on the post-box, and your eyes are simply taking in this external information. You might already know, physically speaking, how your eyes are receiving this colour: the light emitted from the sun hits the post-box and is largely absorbed by the paint, all except light around one particular wavelength. This wavelength, corresponding to the colour of red, is reflected back off the surface of the post-box due to the physical properties of the paint. Some of this light bouncing back will hit your eyes, and this is the moment your eyes receive the physical information from the outside world. But that is only part of the story. The real reason you are *experiencing* the colour red is because the wavelengths hitting the cells at the back of your eye send a message via your optic nerve to a small area at the back of your head, in the occipital lobe of your brain (see Figure 3). When this part of your brain receives the message, its neurons (brain cells) 'fire'. And at that moment only, you experience the colour red. So experiencing the colour is tied to the firing of colour-sensitive neurons in the colour-regions of your brain. These neurons get a message from the eyes and activate, giving you the sensation of redness.

Usually these colour-sensitive neurons in the brain fire when a signal comes in from the eyes, but what if those same neurons fired for another reason? If they fired without the usual signal

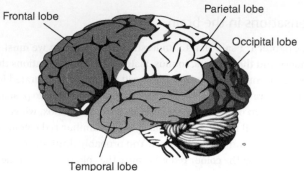

3. The human brain is considered divisible into four lobes: temporal, frontal, parietal, and occipital. These were originally posited as anatomic classifications but are now known to map onto different brain functions. The occipital lobe has a primary visual function, encompassing most of the visual cortex of the brain.

from the eyes we would see red where it simply does not exist in the outside world, in any conventional sense. And this is what happens in synaesthesia: a synaesthete who hears a sound as the colour red is experiencing colours because the colour-centres of his or her brain are firing, but this time with a signal from the ears. Why might this be? Because the pathways that channel signals through the brain appear to be somehow different for synaesthetes. The average brain is set up to allow the colour-centres to fire only when a signal is received from the eyes, but it is possible to imagine a different type of brain where those same neurons receive signals (in some way or other) from the *ears*. In fact if everyone had the brain structure of a synaesthete it would be perfectly natural for us all to think sound was coloured: colour is the firing of a certain part of the brain, and it really does not matter what causes that firing to take place. The resultant experience will be a colour, no matter how those neurons came to be stimulated.

Perhaps this can be best understood by considering that every person—not just synaesthetes—can experience phantom colours under the right conditions. We know this due to the pioneering work of a brain surgeon named Wilder Penfield, whose inventive surgical techniques allowed us to see for the very first time that colours, sounds, smells, tastes, and other sensations derive very firmly from the brain, rather than from the eyes, ears, nose, or other sense organs. Wilder Penfield was an American-Canadian doctor working in the early and middle 20th century on epilepsy patients, and he used a ground-breaking procedure that placed electrodes directly onto the human brain during surgery. Penfield was trying to find the areas responsible for epileptic seizures but was surprised to discover that a whole range of human experiences could be imposed on the patient by gently probing different parts of the brain with an electrode. Patients were given a local anaesthetic only, so were awake while their brains were exposed, and could describe the sensations they were experiencing each time a different part of their brain was probed. Patients reported vivid colours, smells, shapes, and other sensations when different parts of their brains were stimulated. This was a ground-breaking indication that sensations we usually imagine as part of the outside world are in fact tied to clusters of neurons firing in different parts of the brain. This finding, which Wilder Penfield stumbled across somewhat by accident, has given us a powerful way to understand the disconnect between sensations we experience (e.g. colours) and objects that usually stimulate those experiences from the outside world (e.g. post-boxes). Those neurons are *usually* stimulated by the outside objects, but can be stimulated in other ways too. As we will see, contemporary brain scanning of people with synaesthesia gives evidence—and a good explanation—for how these sensations might arise for them.

Seminal studies in the brain imaging of synaesthesia

Historian Jörg Jewanski has combed the historical archives of Germany, France, Italy, Britain, and America to uncover the earliest science writings about synaesthesia, and those earliest

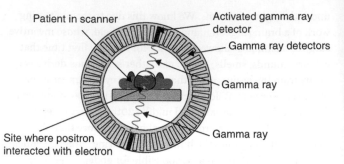

4. PET scanner. Figure shows the detection of gamma rays traced back to the site they were created from the collision of a positron and electron.

studies—now a hundred to two hundred years old—were already speculating on its biological causes. In 1852 the vision expert William White Cooper proposed that the cause of synaesthesia would be found 'not in the eye but in the sensorium', a part of the brain hypothesized to experience sensory information at that time. But it would be another 130 years before the first brain imaging studies could begin to verify this model. In the last thirty years—and the last fifteen years especially—there have been a growing number of studies imaging the brains of synaesthetes, using Positron Emission Tomography (PET), functional Magnetic Resonance Imaging (fMRI), and Diffusion Tensor Imaging (DTI), to name a few (Figure 4).

The first neuroimaging studies of synaesthetes were led by neurologist Richard Cytowic in 1985 and neuroscientist Eraldo Paulesu in 1995. They used techniques that rely on measuring the decay of short-lived radioactive isotopes (or 'tracers') which had been voluntarily ingested by synaesthetes. To understand why synaesthetes would ingest radioactive isotopes, and how this could inform us about synaesthesia, we need to look more closely at the substances themselves and how they allow us to understand the brain. In the PET technique used by Paulesu's team for example, water labelled with isotopes of radioactive oxygen was injected into the bloodstream of synaesthetes. At the same time as receiving the radioactive isotope, the synaesthete volunteers were made to experience synaesthesia (e.g. by being played words that triggered colours). The radiation levels from PET are roughly equivalent to an x-ray, and the tracers very quickly leave the body after testing. But when injected, the tracer can indicate whether any brain region is particularly active (or underactive) at the moment when synaesthesia is being experienced. This is because brain regions that are most active during any given task have higher metabolic demands, and these are the regions where the tracer tends to accumulate. To find out where this is happening, we need to detect their isotopic decay because this decay causes a chain reaction that can be traced back to where in the brain it originated. The decay of the isotope releases a positron which quickly interacts with an electron in the nearby environment to create a pair of gamma rays that travel away from each other. When these gamma rays are detected by sensors around the head, they are picked up at slightly different times and this allows neuroscientists to pinpoint where in the brain they originated from. So the detection of gamma rays allows neuroscientists to infer which parts of the brain were switched on (or switched off) while synaesthetes were being exposed to their synaesthetic triggers and experiencing synaesthesia.

In both 1985 and 1995, synaesthetes' brains showed unusual responses when experiencing synaesthesia. For example, in the 1995 study, word-colour synaesthetes were scanned at the moment they heard words that trigger synaesthetic colours. These synaesthetes were compared to a group of control subjects without synaesthesia (whom we call *non-synaesthetes*) who did the same task. Importantly, synaesthetes' brains showed differences in a number of regions including one called the *posterior inferior temporal cortex*. This region is known to be involved in certain aspects of colour perception, and in linking colour to shape. Although the brains of word-colour synaesthetes were reacting to words differently from the controls' brains, the PET technology of the time was limited in how accurately it could detect or localize any effects. Despite these limitations, early brain studies at the end of the 20th century had given synaesthesia researchers the first indications that synaesthesia could be understood if we looked closely at the human brain—even if we would have to wait a little longer to be certain exactly where and how with greater accuracy.

Within just seven years, synaesthesia scientists had applied a more accurate brain-scanning measure known as fMRI, which can tell us with greater confidence which parts of the brain are working during any given task. fMRI produces detailed images which show bright blobs at different places in the brain. These blobs are the areas that fire or 'light up' to show they are working when the brain is doing any given task—like recalling memories or making decisions, or, indeed, experiencing synaesthetic colours. We can then infer that the areas lighting up are the same areas responsible for the particular brain function of interest. With this technique we could now ask more clearly what parts of the brain are involved when synaesthetes experience synaesthetic sensations. But before we look at the fMRI brain scans of synaesthetes, let us first understand briefly how the brain scanner works and how scientists interpret its data.

The brain scanning takes place while the test-subject is lying down in an MRI scanner—something that looks like a horizontal bed inserted into a large metal donut. This donut is a powerful magnet that gives out a strong magnetic field. In the scanner, the test-subject carries out the mental task of interest, typically by watching something on a screen or listening via headphones. (In a synaesthesia study, the task would be 'having a synaesthetic experience', i.e. the subject might be hearing words or looking at letters on-screen which trigger synaesthetic colours.) The reason we can infer which parts of the brain are used to carry out the task, is because changes in brain activity cause changes in the blood bringing oxygen and glucose (which are needed for metabolism). This change in the blood's oxygenation alters the alignment of molecules within the magnetic field, which can be detected by the scanner. So by looking for changes in oxygenated blood flow we can infer which areas of the brain are working (or 'firing' or 'being activated' or 'lighting up') during different tasks. When fMRI detects differences in the oxygenation of blood, this technique is called *blood oxygenation level-dependent* or BOLD, a technique discovered by Japanese researcher Seiji Ogawa and his team in the early 1990s. They were the first to show that detecting changes in blood oxygenation could be used as a proxy for marking active parts of the brain.

The technique of BOLD contrast as a method of fMRI imaging is used to compare brain activity in one task to some kind of control condition. The control condition is important because it allows us to know exactly what function *in particular* is tied to the area that lights up in the brain. Imagine for example we wanted to understand which parts of the brain process colour in average people. A test-subject is asked to lie in a scanner and look at coloured dots on-screen. This task could cause several areas in their brain to receive oxygenated blood and 'light up' on the fMRI brain scan, but at this point it would be difficult to say whether these were the areas responsible for colour processing in particular. Some areas lighting up might be unrelated to colour altogether, responding instead to the shape of the dots. Or they might not be related to what the subject is seeing at all; the scanner makes loud noises while working so parts of the brain responsible for hearing sounds will have been activated too. In order to be sure that the area we pinpoint is tied to the function we care about, a second task is given with identical properties except for the one detail in question. For example, the control task could have dots that are achromatic (black and white). This allows us to subtract away the working brain areas that are irrelevant, and pinpoint the working brain area we are actually interested in.

Using this type of subtraction technique, neuroscientists have shown, using both fMRI and other techniques (e.g. PET), that one region is particularly at work when average people see colours. This region, towards the back of the head in the occipital lobe, is called human v4 (see Figure 5 in Box 1) and fMRI allows us to take a closer look at what happens to brain area v4 while synaesthetes are experiencing their phantom colours. In 2002, neuroscientist Julia Nunn and her colleagues found that region v4 was more active when word-colour synaesthetes heard words than when they heard beeps. Put differently, when synaesthetes experienced colours (listening to words) their v4 colour region was working much harder than when they saw no synaesthetic colours (listening to beeps). Importantly, this difference was not found in control subjects without synaesthesia: listening to words did not show any extra work being carried out by the colour region v4. A similar finding was reported by Peter Weiss and colleagues for a synaesthete who experienced colours triggered by people's names. Hearing names not only elicited synesthetic colours which could be described by the synaesthete, but also caused brain activity in an area called the *left extra-striate cortex* very near to v4. In another study, neuroscientists Edward Hubbard and V.S. Ramachandran scanned a group of grapheme-colour synaesthetes and controls while they were looking on-screen at graphemes (which again triggered colours for these synaesthetes) or pseudo-graphemes (i.e. nonsense shapes that do not trigger colours). When synaesthetes were viewing true graphemes and so experiencing synaesthetic colours, their brains showed greater modulation of v4 activity compared to when they viewed the pseudo-graphemes. Again this shows that regions normally involved in processing real colours from the outside world appear to be working in the brains of synaesthetes even when there are no colours in the environment.

An alternative explanation for the activation of region v4 in colour-triggering synaesthesia comes from the fact that v4 operates, too, in mental imagery; this area also becomes

Box 1

Figure 5 shows an image created from fMRI brain scanning a grapheme-colour synaesthete (left-hand brain) and a control without synaesthesia (right-hand brain). Brains are shown from the underside, with the front of brains at the bottom of the image and the back of brains at the top. On the left hemisphere of each brain, the white rectangle highlights region (left) v4, shown as a light irregularly bordered shape within each rectangle. (The location and area of v4 was established from earlier scans in which test participants had seen coloured versus achromatic shapes, and this area has been digitally painted onto these scans for illustrative purposes.) On the synaesthete's brain only, there are darker blobs over area v4. These blobs represent brain activity at the moment the scans were taken. V4 usually responds when people are shown colours but there were no colours in the environment—test-subjects were simply reading black graphemes. However, these graphemes triggered synaesthesia for the test-subject on the left, giving the corresponding brain activity in v4. There was no similar activation for the control subject on the right (i.e. no blobs superimposed on v4).

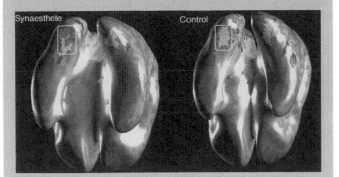

5. Image created from fMRI brain scans of a grapheme-colour synaesthete (left) and a control non-synaesthete (right).

activated when people make colour judgements about greyscale pictures. This leaves open the possibility that synaesthetic colours function not like veridical (real-world) colours but like strong visual images, or indeed like veridical or imagined colours from one synaesthete to the next. (We shall also see below that although v4 has been implicated in a number of imaging studies, it can also be conspicuously absent from one type of synaesthete to the next, or 'light up' on different sides of the brain.)

Two key questions: Functional or structural differences? Direct or indirect connections?

There have been a number of theories about why synaesthesia might be arising in the brains of synaesthetes. These theories take as their starting point the idea that synaesthesia is a type of *co-experiencing* of two different properties—such as a letter-shape and its synaesthetic colour. This co-experiencing might very logically be caused by some type of *cross-communication* (or in neuroscientific terms, *cross-activation*) between the areas responsible for letters and colours respectively: when one area fires up, so does the other. But what kind of brain differences could cause this? In fact, we can tease this apart into two distinct questions: First, do the two areas (e.g. colour and grapheme regions) have more connections between them than in the average brain, or simply the same number of connections but with more free-flow of information? And, second, are these two areas connected directly or are they connected indirectly via some 'middle man' region? There is research supporting both sides of each model and we will review the available evidence below.

Let us start with the first question: Do the brains of synaesthetes have more connections than the average brain, or instead, do they have the same number of connections but with more free-flow of information? This is a key debate among synaesthesia scientists and is often phrased in terms of whether differences in synaesthetes' brains are *structural* or *functional*. A structural difference might mean more dendritic and/or axonal connections than the average person, while a functional difference might mean differences in how freely information can flow down the same number of pathways. To understand this let us imagine driving to London from Town A or Town B, which are an equal distance away. If people from Town A always get to London more reliably it might be because there are more roads from Town A (a structural difference). But alternatively, it might be that there are the same number of roads, but the roads from Town B are always closed for roadworks (a functional difference). This latter is known in neuroscientific terms as *inhibition*—the functional blocking of pathways preventing the free-flow of information. So a structural account would suggest synaesthetes have extra pathways between their centres for graphemes and colours, say. While a functional account would be that all people have exactly the same number of pathways, although these pathways are 'inhibited' in the average person, but 'disinhibited' (i.e. free-flowing) in synaesthetes. If this latter is true, we might all have a 'synaesthetic brain' with multiple connections across different sensory regions, but with pathways that are usually inhibited in the average person.

The disinhibition account of synaesthesia was first proposed by neuroscientists Peter Grossenbacher and Christopher Lovelace, and evidence for their theory comes from the fact that even average people can experience synaesthesia relatively quickly under certain conditions. For example, sound-induced colours have been reported in blind individuals, as little as eight weeks after the onset of blindness. And even average people wearing blindfolds can very quickly come to experience colours triggered by their sense of touch. The speed at which this happens speaks against the idea that people have suddenly grown more connections in their brain to link touch and colour regions. Instead it fits better with the idea that existing connections have simply become 'unmasked' (disinhibited). In one study, a group of average volunteers were blindfolded for five days and were repeatedly fMRI-scanned while performing a number of tasks including touching objects. At the start of the study, the visual regions of the brain were inactive when subjects touched objects but after just five days of blindfolding, there was clear activation in an area of the brain called v1, which usually responds to *visual* stimuli. The sheer speed of this change in revealing 'cross-activation' from touch to vision makes it unlikely that new cortical connections were grown. Moreover, after the blindfolds were removed, this unusual cross-activation fell away rather quickly. So it seems likely that these subjects had existing connections from somatosensory (touch) regions to visual areas that were already present and became somehow unmasked during the five days of blindfolding. Finally, fast-onset synaesthesia might arise from 'psychedelic' drugs like lysergic acid diethylamide (LSD; see Box 2). In some cases these hallucinogens induce relatively fast synaesthetic experiences, for example the onset of colours when listening to music. These drugs, which act on *serotonin* receptors in the brain, have led some neuroscientists such as David Brang and his colleagues to suggest that lifelong (developmental) synaesthesia might be caused by mutations in these same serotonin pathways. Serotonin is a chemical found in blood platelets which acts as a *neurotransmitter* to help relay signals from one part of the brain to another. Any alteration in serotonin pathways might therefore potentially cause a permanent disinhibition in the cross-sensory connections of synaesthetes, similar to the temporary 'unmasking' caused by psychedelic drugs.

Although this paints a compelling picture of rapid disinhibition of existing connections between vision and sound in drug use, and between vision and touch in blindfolding, it is not clear whether this could carry over to developmental synaesthesia in any simple way. Neuroscientists such as Jamie Ward have pointed out that developmental synaesthesias are usually more complex than those in drug-induced synaesthesia (e.g. developmental synaesthesia

Box 2

Transient acquired synaesthesia in drug use has been reported from a range of psychoactive substances, such as mescaline (from the peyote cactus) and the chemical agent psilocybin (derived from fungi known colloquially as 'magic mushrooms') as well as from LSD. LSD was first synthesized by the chemist Albert Hoffman in 1938, but he did not discover its hallucinogenic properties until he accidentally ingested it five years later. When he explored its effects further, his lab notes of 19 April 1943 clearly describe an experience resembling auditory-visual synaesthesia: 'It was particularly striking [after ingesting LSD] how acoustic perceptions such as the noise of a passing auto, the noise of water gushing from the faucet or the spoken word, were transformed in to optical illusions'. Other drugs too, such as ayahuasca (made principally from the Banisteriopsis caapi vine) and MDMA (3,4-methylenedioxy-methamphetamine; commonly known as 'ecstasy') also give rise to experiences that might resemble synaesthesia—or at least enough to merit further inspection. One recent study by neuroscientists David Luke and Devin Terhune looked closely at the link between drug use and synaesthesia-like symptoms across a range of substances. Their systematic review of the science literature showed consistent reporting of cross-sensory experiences in hallucinogenic drug use (e.g. seeing colours while hearing sounds). The nature of these drugs implicates the serotonin system but it is unclear whether the types of sensory experiences elicited resemble true congenital synaesthesia, or not. So while there are reports of colours being triggered by sounds, there is a conspicuous paucity of common synaesthesias such as colours from letters, or time sequences mapped into space. These studies also tended to rely on self-report rather than objective testing, and the single study that has given full details of its attempt to conduct a robust 'test

(continued)

Box 2 Continued

of geniuneness' for grapheme-colour synaesthesia during drug use showed null effects (using a standardized test we will encounter in Chapter 3). It is also difficult to establish a true base-line because participants taking drugs in these studies were already drug users prior to testing. In summary, we are relatively far from understanding the extent to which drug-induced sensations mimic congenital synaesthesia, and exactly whether there are any similarities in a neurological sense. The key hurdle, of course, is that the ethical restrictions on testing for synaesthesia while administering LSD to large numbers of people who have never tried drugs before are (happily!) too prohibitive.

often involves language symbols like letters rather than pure sounds) and so are likely to be formed by different mechanisms. And neuroscientists such as Gary Bargary and Kevin Mitchell point out that irrespective of fast unmasking in drug use or blindfolding, there appear to be distinct borders between different regions of the brain in average people. Although some borders could be 'soft' allowing dormant connections to become disinhibited, it is not well-understood whether synaesthetic regions themselves (e.g. grapheme and colour regions) have borders that are soft or hard. In the latter case there would be no possibility whatsoever of dormant connections in the average person, meaning that synaesthetes would have to have extra connections that non-synaesthetes simply do not have.

Above and beyond the theoretical arguments above, there is some evidence from a different type of brain imaging technique that synaesthetes may in fact have greater connectivity—rather than disinhibited connections—between brain regions. A seminal study by neuroscientists Romke Rouw and Steven Scholte applied the technique of DTI to the study of synaesthetes' brains. To understand what they did and how this showed ground-breaking evidence of structural differences in the brains of synaesthetes, let us first understand the DTI technique.

DTI of synaesthesia

To understand the method of DTI brain imaging, we first have to understand that human brain tissue falls, broadly speaking, into two types—*white matter* and *grey matter*—each made up of different parts of brain cells. Each cell, or neuron, in the brain is typically composed of a cell body, dendrites, and an axon. As Figure 6 shows, dendrites are tree-like structures that emerge

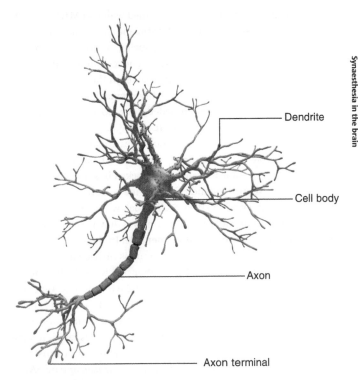

Dendrite

Cell body

Axon

Axon terminal

6. A neuron labelled with its component parts.

from the cell body, and the axon is a long extension which can travel over some distance. These axons (or 'nerve fibres') are surrounded by an electronically insulating layer called myelin, and they function to transmit information from brain cell to brain cell. In this way, axons establish the connectivity between cortical areas, and are what make up white matter in the brain. Grey matter in contrast is the remaining cell body and dendrites. The DTI methodology I will describe below serves to identify bundles of white matter (nerve fibres) in the brain and so highlight the connective capacity of individual brain regions. This capacity can then be compared from one person to the next.

In the DTI technique, the brain is scanned using an MRI scanner, but this time test-subjects simply lie still and do nothing. DTI measures not what the brain is doing during any given task but how it is structured even when resting. The technique relies on detecting the movement of water molecules in the brain, and then uses this movement to infer how the brain must be structured. When water molecules are unimpeded, they move freely in all directions, and this is called *isotropic* (i.e. equal in all directions) movement. However, when water molecules are impeded in some way—for example when they are lying within a cluster of white matter pathways—their movement is blocked in some directions but not others. To understand this, imagine you are throwing a tennis ball down a walled alleyway. The ball will likely ricochet back and forth from wall to wall as it moves down the passage, always restricted by the walls on either side. In the same way, the movement of water molecules in the brain is restricted if they happen to be surrounded by white matter pathways. If the only thing you could see was the movement of the tennis ball you could still infer the presence of the alleyway walls. And so it is in DTI brain imaging: restricted movement of water molecules allows us to infer white matter tracts, and the more the water is restricted the more numerous or robust the surrounding white matter must be. This restricted movement is called *fractional anisotropy* or FA, where greater FA means a greater degree of white matter surrounding the water.

Using this technique, Romke Rouw and Steven Scholte showed that there was greater FA (i.e. more restricted water movement so greater white matter coherence) in the brains of synaesthetes compared to those of control subjects. This difference came exactly where one might expect there to be greater connectivity: in a region called the *inferior temporal cortex* which lies just slightly anterior to the v4 region responsible for colour processing—near to the region that activated in fMRI when synaesthetes had colour experiences from graphemes. The amount of structural difference in this area even corresponded to a measure of the strength of synaesthesia we saw in Chapter 1. *Projector* synaesthetes, who *see* real colours as if they were colours out in space, showed the greatest white matter coherence while *associator* synaesthetes (whose colours are seen only in the mind's eye) showed least. Given this type of evidence from DTI studies, neuroscientists currently tend to talk about greater structural connectivity in the brains of synaesthetes, rather than greater functional disinhibition. However, we might end by considering that different models of synaesthesia need not be mutually exclusive. Neuroscientists such as Edward Hubbard have pointed out that synaesthesia may involve both disinhibition and unusual connectivity, or that different neural theories may explain different types of synaesthesia.

But let us leave for now this question of whether synaesthetes have more actual connections or rather disinhibited connections, and turn instead to the second question we posed above: Do the brains of synaesthetes link the *inducer* (trigger) and *concurrent* (associated sensation) directly or indirectly? Direct connections would mean direct cross-activation from, say, the grapheme region directly to the colour region in the brains of grapheme-colour synaesthetes. Likewise it would mean direct cross-activation from tastes to shapes, from numbers to personalities, and so on for all the different types of synaesthesia we have encountered. This view has become so pervasive in the science literature that the term 'cross-activation' tends to be taken as synonymous for 'direct cross-activation', although there is an alternative hypothesis, that regions might be connected only indirectly. If so, there could be some kind of 'middle man' brain region connected to the inducer and concurrent separately, and playing a type of mediating role between them. One model with this 'indirect' view is the *long-range disinhibited feedback model* proposed by Peter Grossenbacher and Chris Lovelace. This model suggests that incoming information from the trigger (e.g. letter) is first received in the brain at the appropriate place (e.g. the letter processing brain region). This information is then fed to a 'middle man' region to serve some normal purpose in processing the stimulus (e.g. integrating it with other information from the environment). But once received by the 'middle man', the information bounces back unexpectedly to an unusual areas such as colour or taste. Their model suggests that these *feedback connections* are usually inhibited in most people but are *dis*inhibited in synaesthetes. So this particular indirect model of connectivity happens to also favour a disinhibition account.

Other feedback models such as the *re-entrant processing model for grapheme-colour synaesthesia* are agnostic about whether feedback is from extra connections or disinhibited connections, and different models also name a number of potential middle-man regions. Perhaps the most notable is an area known as the *binding* region, located in the parietal cortex (see Figure 3). 'Binding' is a normal process which allows all humans to tie together information from different senses. So when we see a red apple, its colour and shape are processed in different parts of the brain, but are integrated by a third region which 'binds' shape and colour together. Binding ensures we see an integrated red apple, rather than the potentially alarming impression of a patch of redness floating in space somewhere *other* than on top of where we perceive the apple's shape. The *hyperbinding* model of synaesthesia proposed by Lynn Robertson and colleagues suggests that synaesthesia could arise through over-activation of binding mechanisms in the parietal lobe. This would lead to unusual binding between colours and letters, or between tastes and words, and so on. Her model is particularly compelling because the parietal lobe is also implicated by neuroimaging studies. Synaesthetes' parietal regions have been shown to be active in fMRI studies during synaesthetic experiences, and also show connectivity differences in DTI (i.e. greater FA). And synaesthetes' parietal regions also show thicker grey matter as well as evidence of being more integrated to other brain systems. A Swiss team led by Jürgen Hänggi looked at regions where the cortex matches in thickness, in order to infer connectivity between them. They found that the parietal region of synaesthetes appears to act as a hub to many other brain regions, again implicating it in synaesthetic experiences. Similarly, functional connectivity analyses of grapheme-colour synaesthetes by Christopher Sinke and colleagues reveal increased connectivity between parietal and visual areas. But whether its role is in binding functions—or indeed other functions of the parietal cortex like paying attention—we can only speculate.

Gary Bargary and Kevin Mitchell have suggested that although parietal regions likely play a role in synaesthesia, the connections between the inducer and concurrent may still be direct. They point to a striking principle of cortical connectivity more generally, which is *small world design*, meaning that the majority of connections in the human brain are between areas that are close together. Similarly, Edward Hubbard and colleagues have pointed out that one of the most common forms of synaesthesia—grapheme-colour synaesthesia—happens to link two properties (letters and colours) that are processed in neighbouring brain regions. This idea of adjacency is wrapped up in the notion that grapheme and colour regions should therefore connect *directly*, rather than over longer distances via a 'middle man'. But one recent study by Tessa van Leeuwen and her team suggests that communication between the synaesthetic trigger and its concurrent might vary between direct or indirect from one synaesthete to the next. Van Leeuwen measured functional connectivity in the brains of grapheme-colour synaesthetes and found that the best model for projectors (whose colours are seen out in space) was of a direct cross-activation between regions processing the inducer and concurrent, while for associators (whose colours are seen in the mind's eye) it was of indirect cross-activation via the parietal cortex. So the parietal lobe—although not a sensory region itself—may play a vital role in the binding of sensations in some synaesthetes, although perhaps not all.

A critical consideration of neuroscientific studies

As imaging techniques develop, we will have a yet clearer understanding of how synaesthesia arises in the brain, but we should acknowledge current limitations in the field. The picture I have painted above from DTI studies of white matter has an elegant ring. Researchers have suggested synaesthetes have 'extra' sensations like colours because they have 'extra' connective brain pathways near to colour-regions. But it is important to not over-simplify. Greater FA (restricted water movement) in DTI studies is often interpreted as showing 'more white matter connections' in the brains of synaesthetes, but neuroscientists Bargary and Mitchell point out that the microstructural correlates of DTI findings are actually poorly understood. Movement of water molecules can be influenced not only by the *number* of axons in a tract, but also by their diameter, by how they line up in a specific direction, by the degree to which they are bundled, and by other cellular parameters such as the amount of myelination (the electronically insulating layer surrounding the axon). So it is safer to describe DTI findings as showing the *structural integrity* of the white matter, rather than simply the *number* of pathways. And even the direction of results requires clarification. Studies tend to emphasize their findings of *greater* FA (i.e. *greater* white matter integrity) in synaesthetes. This fits intuitively with the notion that synaesthetes have additional sensations compared to the average person. But a closer inspection of results shows that many studies also find *reduced* FA in some parts of synaesthetes' brains (i.e. under-connectivity or reduced coherence of white matter). For example, my own study with Marie Rehme and colleagues found reduced white matter coherence within the corpus callosum of sequence-personality synaesthetes (whose letters and numbers have synaesthetic personalities). This is a region that links the left and right hemispheres of the brain but also plays a role in social understanding. And other studies too show a mixture of both greater and lesser FA—so *altered* connectivity rather than exclusively *increased* connectivity—from one form of synaesthesia to the next, and even within individual synaesthetes.

Another interesting inconsistency is the extent to which synaesthesia can be seen on the left or right side of the brain. The grapheme area is usually lateralized on the left side of the brain, but structural differences in seminal DTI studies of grapheme-colour synaesthetes were found near colour regions on the right side of the brain. And there is inconsistency, too, in the number of areas implicated, since studies have found white and grey matter differences not only near colour regions but also thicker grey matter in motor/pre-motor regions usually responsible for movement, and differing connectivity in prefrontal regions of the brain sometimes involved in cognitive control—to name a few. Synaesthetes may therefore have widespread brain differences, the causes of which are still poorly understood.

One recent review by neuroscientists Jean-Michel Hupé and Michel Dojat closely inspected the methods and assumptions of synaesthesia brain imaging studies and concluded that many are statistically underpowered, and that a surprising number find no evidence for any involvement of colour regions at all. They point out that v4 activation by synaesthetic colours had only been found in five out of twelve previous fMRI investigations, and their own fMRI study again found no evidence of overlap between brain regions for real colours and synaesthetic colours. One explanation may come from differences among grapheme-colour synaesthetes themselves. Van Praag and colleagues have shown that BOLD responses in the colour-selective v4 region is different for different grapheme-colour synaesthetes, being found especially for synaesthetes with highly automatic colours (in left v4) or colours that appear in specific spatial locations (in left and right v4). These results may go some way towards explaining differences in v4 involvement across different synaesthesia studies. But what seems clear from careful reviews such as that of Hupé and Dojat, is that we have a core problem in that studies tend to scan only small numbers of synaesthetes. Small numbers mean we are limited in the statistical conclusions we can draw from each investigation. But small numbers happen to be the natural result of difficulties in recruiting subjects, given the rarity of synaesthesia. Happily, the unifying influence of the world wide web means we can now reach out to more synaesthetes than ever before. This fact, combined with the slowly reducing costs of brain imaging, means that future studies can gain greater power by scanning more test-subjects with more accurate measures.

Chapter 3
Synaesthesia and the arts

As I write this chapter I am listening to one of my favourite
pieces of piano music. It is called 'Blue Pacific', played by Hana
Chu and written by the American composer Michael Torke.
It is safe the say that were it not for synaesthesia, this piece of
music would not exist. Michael Torke is a synaesthete and this
music was written—in part—as a reflection of his synaesthetic
colours from playing and hearing musical notes. The piece has
an expressive melody that develops around the key of D major
which, in Michael's synaesthesia, is a bright and rich blue.
So the name of this piece is more than just a description of the
ocean: it is also the synaesthetic colour of the musical key that
was adapted so beautifully when Michael Torke wrote this piece.
In this chapter and Chapter 4, I will consider the link between
synaesthesia, art, and creativity. Some key scientific questions
we will encounter relate to whether there is an intrinsic beauty
in the artwork created by synaesthetes which could make it
inherently attractive to all people. We will ask whether synaesthetes
are able to tap into aesthetic beauty in some kind of privileged way.
And we will ask, too, whether synaesthetes are more creative
than the average person, and whether they engage more often
in artistic pursuits.

Who are the famous synaesthete artists?

Anyone reading a chapter about synaesthesia and the arts might first ask one question in particular: Who are the famous synaesthetes in art and culture? This is a natural question not only because artists, celebrities, and other famous people can now reach us by more creative media than ever before, and not only because there is a contemporary curiosity about aspects of their lives. But I believe we also have an interest in putting a face to synaesthesia, so we can understand who might be experiencing the unusual sensations that seem so very different to our own. But a more interesting story will be to explain to you why it is particularly *not* possible to provide a straightforward list of famous synaesthetes. This is because there are several facts about synaesthesia that converge on two truths: that those who say they are synaesthetes may not be, and that those who are true synaesthetes may not say so. More confusing still, is that the one place we would expect to find many synaesthetes (which we will see is in the creative world of the arts) is precisely the place we would also find many people reporting synaesthesia who are not synaesthetes at all. So let's unpack this riddle below.

There are many famous people who have described having synaesthesia or synaesthesia-like experiences. And there are many journalists, bloggers, vloggers, and other commentators who have attributed synaesthesia to others. The internet is full of such claims, as are magazines, newspapers, and other media sources. *Wikipedia* for example provides a list of over twenty people it declares to be synaesthetes, and these individuals range from classical composers (Olivier Messiaen: coloured sounds) to contemporary musicians (Pharrell Williams: coloured sounds), to authors (Vladimir Nabokov: coloured letters), to scientists (Richard Feynman: coloured letters), to painters (Wassily Kandinsky: coloured sounds or noisy vision), and so on. But how confident can we be about these claims, and why might we want to take time to examine them carefully? Remarkably, empirical studies have shown that for every one true synaesthete who claims to have synaesthesia, there are around five *non*-synaesthetes who claim to have synaesthesia. In other words, somebody claiming to have synaesthesia is still roughly five times more likely *not* to be a synaesthete than to actually be one. Scientists can only know for sure who the true synaesthetes are by running a diagnostic test. So unless members of any 'famous synaesthete list' have been tested, it is difficult for an outsider to conclude either way, because synaesthesia cannot be confirmed from self-declaration alone and it cannot easily be attributed to other people without careful testing.

In 2005, my colleague Jamie Ward and I tried to find out how common synaesthesia was in the population. We ran a study in which we individually screened 1,500 people for synaesthesia. We tested 1,000 of them for grapheme-colour synaesthesia (i.e. coloured letters or numbers) and we tested the remaining 500 people for a wider range of 128 different synaesthetic types. For the 500 people we tested most comprehensively, we first asked one very important question: we asked them whether *they* thought they had synaesthesia. We carefully explained exactly what synaesthesia was, and we gave them many examples of different types of synaesthesia. Then we showed them all the types of synaesthesia we were testing for, and we simply asked them to tell us whether they thought they had any. From the 500 people we asked, around 120 said they believed they had a type of synaesthesia. But when we gave them an objective test to find out for sure who the synaesthetes really were, we found only twenty-two genuine cases. This came as a great surprise—that so many people would claim to have synaesthesia even when we had made efforts to be absolutely certain we had explained what synaesthesia was. And there was a reverse to this too, perhaps even more surprising. Not only did a large number of non-synaesthetes claim to have synaesthesia, but most of the *true* synaesthetes did not realize they were synaesthetes at all—and many just assumed they were not. Many of these true synaesthetes simply thought that all people experienced the world the way they did, so had never mentioned it to anyone before our testing. They expressed great surprise to learn they were different to the average person and even found it hard to believe. So all this research led to two surprising conclusions: those who say they are synaesthetes may not be, and those who are synaesthetes may not say so.

So why are many people without synaesthesia keen to claim they have it? In our study, a large group were self-confessed 'malingers' who initially claimed to fit the description of synaesthesia, but then subsequently retracted their claims in full when asked again at a later date. The reasons for this may be complex, but there could be an element of 'social desirability'—when people answer questions in studies and surveys, they tend to do so in a way that will be viewed favourably by others. Since synaesthesia might be considered interesting, there could be a tendency for people to want to claim they have it. Also, there was another group of individuals who claimed to have synaesthesia, but just because they misunderstood the very nature of synaesthesia itself, despite our careful descriptions. Importantly, these people were often artists who reasonably mistook synaesthesia for their heightened appreciation of colour, or for their artistic ability to creatively (but deliberately) combine sensations in unusual ways in their artwork. As we will discuss later, all people can make pairings across the senses in ways that feel intuitively 'just right'—colours with sounds, tastes with shapes, and so on. For example, it might feel 'just right' for all people to think of an uplifting piece of music as being bright yellow rather than murky purple. But this type of deliberate association is not synaesthesia. It is just part of the normal ability in all people to pair the senses in preferred ways. So there is a fine line here, but an important difference, between someone (not a synaesthete) saying that a joyful song is yellow, and someone (a synaesthete) who genuinely perceives a specific shade of yellow every time he or she hears that song. The true developmental synaesthetes will have done so since they were young, and would have a complex range of different sound-colour pairings that always appear automatically, without effort, and consistently over time—all traits which we have described earlier as being key indicators of synaesthesia.

But we now hit a paradox which is that although artists are people perhaps likely to think they have synaesthesia by mistake, they are also the people most likely to be synaesthetes as genuine cases. In the pages that follow we will see that having synaesthesia brings a creative streak to the personality, and that synaesthetes are significantly more likely to follow artistic careers than the average person. Synaesthesia can contribute to the creation of beautiful artwork, and synaesthetes do tend to be artists more often than the average person. Studies have shown that synaesthetes tend to spend more time engaged in creative activities, and especially creative activities tied to their synaesthesia. So synaesthetes with coloured music, for example, are more likely to play an instrument than other people.

In summary, we would expect to find a large proportion of people incorrectly claiming to have synaesthesia in artistic circles (because they mistake synaesthesia for artistic sentiment), but conversely, artistic circles are also places where true synaesthetes will be found in larger numbers than elsewhere. This means that scientists must take great care to ensure that the studies they run on people with synaesthesia have actually recruited genuine synaesthetes—rather than anyone mistaking themselves for a synaesthete in error. To achieve this we run a simple diagnostic test, which is described further below. But although it requires testing for me to verify genuine synaesthesia, I want to point out that it is important for true synaesthetes to be believed. And I know this more than most: I have examined the experiences of thousands of synaesthetes, both adults and children, and I have known cases of synaesthetes who have been met with disbelief, derision, or even reprimand when expressing simple descriptions of their perceptual worlds. In one recent science report, simple synaesthesia was even mistaken for schizophrenia, although happily, such misdiagnoses are rare. But I have spent my academic career trying to remove the mystery surrounding synaesthesia so that synaesthetes can be believed and better understood—in society, the media, schools, universities, and anywhere else. All the famous people I have chosen to name in this chapter seem to me like very reasonable candidates as genuine synaesthetes, which is why I chose them in particular. I have made no mention about 'famous synaesthetes' who I suspect might *not* have synaesthesia because I am not here to say who isn't a synaesthete. I have just taken time to explain why it is difficult for even a synaesthesia scholar to be sure, given these few surprising facts about synaesthesia itself.

The artistic allure for synaesthetes

As discussed, there is a certain type of circularity when finding high rates of synaesthesia among artists: there is more genuine synaesthesia for artists, but also more reporting of synaesthesia in error. This circularity can best be summed up by a study carried out by George Domino in 1989. Domino surveyed 358 fine art students and found that 23 per cent reported synaesthesia—a rate that is very high compared to that of 4 per cent for the general population. But Domino did not administer any diagnostic tests to verify who the true synaesthetes were—he simply took their self-reports as accurate. Given that artists sometimes confuse synaesthesia with artistic sensibility, this self-report methodology would have artificially inflated the number of synaesthetes in his set of art students. And this was confirmed thirty years later. A team lead by Nicolas Rothen in 2010 repeated the study but this time *did* use a robust diagnostic test for synaesthesia. Rothen found the true rate of synaesthesia in art students was around 15 per cent. (I have had to scale this number so we can compare the two studies directly for the types of synaesthesia they were looking for.) These two studies therefore support what we have already encountered: that synaesthesia is over-reported by artists (the true prevalence is not 23 per cent but only 15 per cent) but that their rates of synaesthesia are still far higher than the 4 per cent found in the general population. So what is it that draws synaesthetes to the world of creativity and art?

In Chapter 1 I described Sean Day, a synaesthete with coloured music who seems to have been drawn towards music as a result of his synaesthesia. As a boy, Sean realized that the timbres of different musical instruments each had their own rich colours—and still do today: piano is blue, violin is brown, and so on. Sean believes this gave him a particular penchant to explore music that he otherwise might not have had, and he has certainly become an accomplished pianist. I once heard him play piano in a splendid marble town hall in Spain, and I wondered how exactly his synaesthesia had affected his desire to play music. Sean described this to me recently in his own words:

> My synaesthesia inspired me to teach myself all I could. I started my music training on organ (which makes me see a sort of mother-of-pearl on a polished gold background) but I sought out the piano because of the sky blue cyan colour it produced. And synaesthesia also led me to electric guitars, bright reds, oranges, and pinks, which I went after during my teenage years. In contrast, bowed string instruments are nice enough—all brown, but 'normal'. But it was definitely the synaesthetic colours that led me to my all-time favourite instrument to play: the vibraphone—gorgeous shades of purple in its timbre—which I played for a few years in a high school jazz band.

So even as a teenager Sean Day had already been drawn to multiple instruments, intrigued by their colours, with his synaesthesia inspiring him to try to develop talent. But does synaesthesia also play a role in how synaesthetes might compose particular pieces? To understand this we need to explore further the sensations of music synaesthetes, and how these can come to play a role in the creation of artwork.

Let us return to the piano piece *Blue Pacific*, which is still playing through the speakers in my office. How exactly was this music created, and what qualities of synaesthesia can be found in it? Whereas Sean Day describes the colours of instruments according to their timbre, the composer Michael Torke realized as a young boy that he had colours from musical keys, or sometimes pitches. As he grew older Michael began composing professionally and wrote a series of pieces for orchestra named after colours. These early pieces were composed within a given key, and named appropriately for his synaesthesia: *Ecstatic Orange* (1984–5), *Bright Blue Music* (1985), *Green* (1986), *Purple* (1987), and *Ash* (1988). So his *Green* symphony, for example, is built around his key of green E major. Later, Torke returned to this theme in writing *Blue Pacific* around his D major key of blue. As I listen to it, I am struck by the fact that even to a non-synaesthete, the music *Blue Pacific* does feel 'blue-coloured'. Of course the photo-cover shows a serene body of blue water, and the music cleverly evokes the flawless ebb and flow of the sea. But perhaps there is also something fitting to me about Michael's blue D major? We will see later in this book that non-synaesthetes *do* have the ability to intuitively feel the 'rightness' of synaesthetes' associations, but of course Michael Torke has a link between sound and music that I cannot share at any phenomenological level. Like most synaesthetes, he has very certain colour associations, so let us explore next how specific these colours are, how can we measure them, and how exactly they are used in synaesthetic artworks.

The diagnostic test for synaesthesia

Like all synaesthetes, Michael Torke describes his synaesthetic colours in depth and detail. In an interview he gave to *Performance Today* on public radio, Michael Torke labelled his colour for E major as

> a kind of a spring green, very very warm. E minor gets slightly more blue added to it. But it is not a blue green, just a colder green.

G major is yellow. Whereas G minor gets to be kind of a burnt yellow
or an ochre. G-sharp which is the third scale degree of E Major...is
green, but if I isolate g-sharp, that becomes this almost kind of
pumpkin orange. So G-sharp Major would have that kind of sound.

These descriptions show a depth of detail when synaesthetes
describe their experiences. Just this morning I asked a synaesthete
the colour of 'Friday' within his colourful synaesthetic week. 'It is a
lemon yellow' he said,

> but it is a very specific shade. It's the same lemon yellow as a
> Lacoste polo sport shirt I had from the late 1980s, probably...1987.
> It had a very specific lemon yellow shade and it's the only time I've
> ever seen it. That's Friday.

So synaesthetes' descriptions are rich in colour and complexity, so
much so that they will often go to great lengths trying to describe
them. In my research lab in the UK we devise computerized tests
that allow synaesthetes to show us their synaesthetic colours
on-screen, by picking them from an extensive electronic colour
palette. During our test we present synaesthetes with the inducers
of their synaesthesia—say, a letter or number—and we ask them
to choose from the palette to show us the synaesthetic colours
these evoke. Synaesthetes often spend large amounts of time
finding exactly the shade they need because they have a highly
specific notion of exactly what that colour should be. And when
synaesthetes choose their colours from this palette they do so
in a very specific way which, importantly, allows us to diagnose
synaesthesia. We mentioned in Chapter 1 that a key trait
separating synaesthetes from non-synaesthetes is *consistency over
time*. This means that synaesthetes' colours (or tastes, or smells, or
shapes, etc.) do not change in any major way from one day to the
next. If the letter A happens to be red for any given synaesthete,
it will always tend to be red for that same synaesthete. If the word
'society' happens to taste of onions, it will always taste of onions.
And this consistency over time can be measured to diagnose

synaesthesia. During the diagnostic test, we show inducers on screen one at a time—for example we show the letters A to Z. The test-subject matches a colour to each letter, for example he or she might select a very specific shade of green for the letter E. Then we show the letters again in a surprise retest and ask the synaesthete to repeat the task. Finally, we examine the first and second presentation of each letter for how consistent its colour was. A synaesthete is highly consistent over time—he or she might select the same specific shade of green each time on seeing the letter E. On the other hand, people *without* synaesthesia will be largely inventing their colour associations, so by the time they have seen all twenty-six letters it would be hard to remember which colour was which. This means that non-synaesthetes are not very consistent when shown the same letter twice—they choose different colours over time. And this is the basis of the diagnostic test: synaesthetes are consistent and non-synaesthetes are less consistent, and this is how we separate genuine synaesthetes from the pack.

This feature of consistency over time can be quantified numerically because every colour in our electronic colour palette has a number value to represent its exact shade. This number quantifies how light the colour is, how saturated it is, and exactly what hue it has. The two colours selected by a synaesthete for any given letter presented twice will be very close in number. This allows us to quantify synaesthetic consistency as small differences in colour distance for synaesthetes (because they choose similar colours over time) and large differences for non-synaesthetes (because they choose colours that are different). And the same principle of consistency can be used to diagnose many different forms of synaesthesia. Figure 7 and Box 3 shows the testing interface we have devised to screen for another type of synaesthesia, lexical-gustatory synaesthesia, by presenting trigger words on-screen to induce their synaesthetic flavours in the mouth. Once the flavour is triggered, the synaesthete can describe his or her experience using the taste-selection pie chart

Box 3

Figure 7 shows a screen shot from the diagnostic test for lexical-gustatory synaesthesia I have devised with colleagues Alberta Ipser and James Hughes. During the test, a target word is shown on the left (here, the word 'question'). This word triggers a synaesthetic flavour which the synaesthete describes using the taste-selection pie chart on the right. The synaesthete adjusts the segments of the pie chart to indicate his or her synaesthetic flavour in terms of its five taste dimensions (sweet, salty, sour, bitter, umami). For example if a participant associated the word 'question' with the flavour of a cheeseburger, he or she might sense it as mostly umami (i.e. meaty), then salty, a bit sweet, and then a bit sour from the relish. The taste will not be bitter at all, unless the burger was burnt. The synaesthete would then adjust the pie chart accordingly, making umami the largest segment, then salt, and so on. The 'No Taste' button allows for certain words which may have no synaesthetic

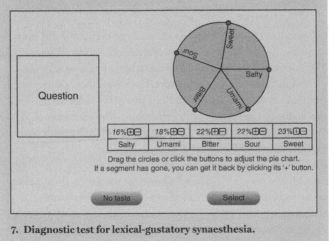

7. Diagnostic test for lexical-gustatory synaesthesia.

(*continued*)

Box 3 Continued

experience. Each word is presented twice during the test and this allows us to calculate how consistently the synaesthete described the tastes for each word. We convert this consistency to a percentage, and have found that it is an excellent diagnostic for lexical-gustatory synaesthesia (with this evaluation coming from a statistical measures that assesses how well diagnostics can separate synaesthetes from controls). Our test is so difficult for non-synaesthetes that virtually all score less than around 25 per cent. In contrast, over 90 per cent of synaesthetes score above this threshold.

on the right. We can then quantify the synaesthetic flavour in terms of its five taste dimensions (sweet, salty, sour, bitter, umami). Just as in the colour test, each trigger word is presented twice so we can calculate how consistently the synaesthete reports the synaesthetic flavour.

So synaesthetic experiences are consistent over time and they also have a depth of quality that is alive to the synaesthete. The colour palette we show to synaesthetes has over sixteen million different shades of colours, but synaesthetes sometimes complain it still cannot match their internal world. Sometimes this is due to the limits of our technology—we cannot easily show metallic tints or iridescence on our computerized screen. We cannot show colours that are 'both purple and yellow at the same time', as one synaesthete described a colour she was searching for. Other synaesthetes complain we cannot match the vibrancy or the intensity, or the added texture or glint or radiance. So there are clearly scientific limitations in our testing. But even if synaesthetes feel sometimes unhappy with the choices available to them, they nonetheless hone in on the closest colour, and show themselves to be consistent over time. This consistency and detail is also true of synaesthetic tastes, synaesthetic shapes, synaesthetic textures, and all types of synaesthetic associations we have tested.

Synaesthete artists and synaesthetic art

The depth, detail, texture, and vibrancy of synaesthetic sensations is perhaps one reason why artists with synaesthesia have drawn on them to create compelling pieces of artwork. Synaesthetes have conveyed their synaesthetic experiences in different forms of music, painting, dance, literature, abstract composition, sculpture, and more. One of my favourite pieces of synaesthetic art is the painting *Clouds Rise Up* (2004) by artist and synaesthete Carol Steen. I saw it in person at the exhibition *Synesthesia: Art and the Mind* at the McMaster Museum of Art, Ontario, Canada in 2008, where it sat alongside artwork from David Hockney, Joan Mitchell, Marcia Smilack, Charles Burchfield, Tom Thomson, Wassily Kandinsky, and Vincent Van Gogh. (All of these artists have exploited visual qualities evocative of synaesthesia; some are confirmed synaesthetes like Carol Steen or the fascinating photographic artist Marcia Smilack; others like Wassily Kandinsky are very likely to have been synaesthetes; while others still may not be synaesthetes at all but simply use synaesthetic techniques with artistic licence.) Carol Steen's painting *Clouds Rise Up* is modest in size but an explosion of vibrancy. The background is a mixed shade of forest green with a luminescent quality that makes it shine. And layered on top are vibrant, jaunty, streaks of red and orange which pop out from the background and dance over the canvas. The picture represents an experience of synaesthesia that presented itself to Carol Steen one day while she was listening to a musician playing the Shakuhachi flute. This Japanese instrument has a lilting quality and was being played at a slow tempo when it triggered Steen's synaesthesia. Each note the musician played seemed to have two sounds, and so it produced two synaesthetic colours: the red and the orange that move together across the canvas. The green background to the painting references the colour of the flute itself, a shade of khaki-forest metallic green. Carol Steen named her painting *Clouds Rise Up* because this is what she saw as she listened to the musician play his flute. But although her aim was to capture the beauty of that one transient moment into a permanent representation in oil paints, there is also an element of artistic freedom in her work. Because importantly, the *extent* to which art mirrors synaesthesia can vary from painting to painting, and from artist to artist.

Timothy B. Layden is another widely appreciated artist and synaesthete, and he describes synaesthesia as taking a particularly prominent role in his recent compositions. Layden experiences synaesthetic shapes and colours when hearing sounds, and his series *The Shape of Sounds* is a combination of research, sound, and visual artwork in which synaesthesia takes centre stage. Layden starts his artistic process by capturing 'soundscapes'. Here he first seeks out or generates sounds to trigger interesting synaesthetic perceptions, then records those sounds to edit. When editing, Layden explores the sounds to find elements of shape he finds enjoyable or beautiful. The resultant soundscapes combine these sounds while digitally emphasizing or uniting different elements. Layden then begins to draw or paint sketches of the coloured shapes he hears. Finally, he unites these pictorial elements into a larger artwork, using artistic freedom to bring together the different visual elements in a single pictorial composition. *The Shape of Sounds* series comprises twenty-two paintings, thirty-three drawings, and eleven soundscapes, and *Dark Glistening* is an example from the series shown in Figure 8. Many pieces in this series are highly colourful but *Dark Glistening* is predominantly achromatic with a hint of yellow in the haze-like band across the centre. (This painting can be viewed while listening to the soundscape upon which it is based at http://theshapeofsounds.com) I find Layden's work beautiful and complex, but also intriguing, not only in how he fashions individual shapes into larger compositions, but also in the range

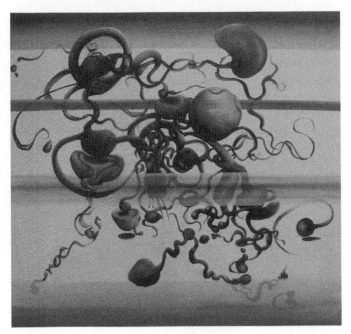

8. *Dark Glistening* by Timothy B. Layden; 1 m × 1 m mixed media on canvas.

of shapes he experiences from synaesthesia and the ways in which shapes link to colours and sounds. Layden himself has spent considerable time with fellow artist Christine Söffing looking for similarities across their synaesthesias and finding hidden links between them. (Some of his shapes are strikingly similar to those of Söffing shown in Figure 1 at the start of this book, and we will discuss why this might be in Chapter 5.)

We hinted above that different artists can use synaesthesia more or less in their work. Some synaesthetic artists do not use synaesthesia in their professional life at all, while others place it to the fore. And even *non*-synaesthete artists might overtly use synaesthesia as a device. The artist David Hockney is reported to have used synaesthesia-like associations when designing opera stage sets, inspired by the musical scores. But synaesthesia is not obviously apparently in his other works (and it is unclear to me whether he self-declares as a synaesthete or not). Even if synaesthesia *is* used by synaesthetic artists, the artwork does not automatically become a literal depiction. Many synaesthete artists describe their synaesthesia as a starting point, like a jumping board from which to leap into artistic creativity. But if synaesthetes *do* choose to exploit their synaesthesia in art forms, how will this art be received? Is synaesthesia aesthetically appealing to people without synaesthesia? Put simply, does synaesthesia make for 'good art'?

How universal is synaesthetic art?

We saw above that Michael Torke wrote a number of musical scores named after the synaesthetic colours they produced. But he has also emphasized that synaesthesia is just one small part of his musical process and he has voiced a concern that too much focus on his subjective synaesthesia might hinder his artistic desire to express something universal. After all, how could something so individual to a synaesthete be used as a framework to produce something with a universal truth? In actuality, Michael Torke need not worry; evidence has shown that art founded on synaesthetic sensations is inherently pleasing to all people. In other words, the subjective synaesthetic experiences of Michael Torke and other synaesthetes have a universal quality that aesthetically appeals to everyone.

In 2008, a team of researchers led by Jamie Ward worked with animator Samantha Moore to look at how synaesthesia might be judged by audiences. Ward and Moore were asking whether non-synaesthetes would appreciate synaesthesia as a form of art, and if it might be aesthetically pleasing when judged by an audience. They first interviewed a group of synaesthetes who perceived colours in music. Animator Samantha Moore played them a range of different notes at varying pitches and timbres, and used their descriptions of synaesthesia to create short animated clips—each one showing the synaesthetic colours, shapes, and movements triggered by the various sounds. Moore animated a hundred different audio-visual clips in total, and I have given some examples in Figure 9 and Box 4. Each animation represented a true snapshot of synaesthesia, by showing a colourful, often moving shape, presented along with the sound that had triggered it (e.g. a yellow zigzag moving rightwards, to the sound of a violin playing D sharp). And then the researchers did something interesting: they took each audio-visual clip and modified the visuals in a subtle way. They changed the colour, or rotated its orientation by 90 degrees. Or they swapped the audio between two different clips. In the end, Moore had created a hundred clips of true synaesthesia, and a hundred modified clips. The researchers then played all the clips to an audience of people without synaesthesia, who just listened and watched. The audience did not know what they were watching but were simply asked to decide which clips they liked best, in an aesthetic sense. To be clear, they were not asked to judge whether the sounds and images fitted together, but simply whether they liked the clip or not. And the results showed that audiences preferred the true clips from synaesthetes. In other words, synaesthetic experiences, when represented as artwork and shown to audiences, are intuitively judged as aesthetically pleasing. So all this means that when Michael Torke, Timothy B. Layden, and others use their synaesthesia as a backbone to their artwork, they are producing something of universal beauty which is likely to give aesthetic pleasure to their audiences.

In Chapter 4 we will see two more traits that link synaesthesia and art. We will learn that synaesthetes are objectively more creative than the average person, and have certain personality traits linked to heightened imagination. Synaesthetes also have specific visual benefits, such as the ability to better distinguish facial features and their expressions (a useful skill for portrait artists). These

Box 4

Figure 9 shows screen captures of moving audio-visual clips created by animator Samantha Moore for a study. These animations represented the synaesthetic shapes, colours, and textures triggered by sounds for five different synaesthetes. There were a hundred animations in total, and four examples are shown in screen-shot here, triggered by the following sounds: a single cello string bowed (images 1 and 4); two cello notes bowed simultaneously representing an octave (image 2) or a musical fifth (image 3). In the original animations, colours for shapes/backgrounds were (for images 1–4 respectively): brown/grey, indigo/white, indigo/white, grey/brown. The original animations also capture the movement and morphing of shapes in response to the dynamic qualities of the sound. In the examples here, shapes moved from left to right (images 1 and 3), from right to left (image 4), or from bottom to top (image 2). In addition to these hundred true animations (i.e. representative of

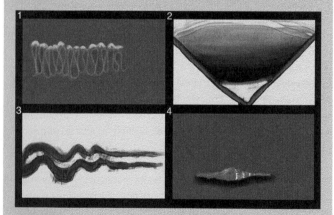

9. Screenshots from an animation showing the shapes of sounds, described by synaesthetes and animated by Samantha Moore.

synaesthetic experiences) Moore created a hundred more which switched colour (e.g. presenting image 3 in brown not blue), switched direction (e.g. presenting image 4 moving left to right), or switched sound (e.g. presenting the visuals of image 1 with the sound of image 2). Naïve participants rated the original unadulterated animations as more aesthetically pleasing.

differences are just one of a number of ways we will see in which synaesthetes can differ from the average person. And by considering both advantages and disadvantages, we will ask whether synaesthesia might be viewed as a 'gift' or a 'condition'.

Chapter 4
Is synaesthesia a 'gift' or a 'condition'?

Ever since scientists first learned about the remarkable tastes, colours, sounds, and other sensations of synaesthesia we have wondered how these experiences might affect synaesthetes themselves. Is there a consequence to having synaesthesia, even beyond the obvious difference of experiencing merged sensations? Do synaesthetes have qualities that make them different to non-synaesthetes in other ways? Do they show differences in everyday abilities like memory, mental calculation, general perception, creative thinking, use-of-language, and so on? Are these differences 'gifts' that make synaesthetes rise above the masses? Or are there also disadvantages to being a synaesthete? In this chapter we will leave aside the unusual sensory experiences that define synaesthesia and look instead at synaesthetes themselves.

Are synaesthetes more creative?

In Chapter 3 we saw that synaesthetes follow careers in the arts more often than the average person and one obvious explanation is that synaesthesia can provide interesting subject matter—perhaps a fascinating synaesthetic shape to paint. It might also be the case that synaesthesia entices artists towards their medium, as when musical instruments become appealing for the attractive synaesthetic colours they can produce. But synaesthesia can also play a different role for artists—independent of synaesthetic sensations themselves. We will see in this section that synaesthetes may be inherently more *creative* than the average person, even independently of synaesthesia itself.

We can think of 'creativity' as the ability to pair together thoughts and ideas in ways that stand out from mundane convention. Or as the ability to find innovative links hidden in the everyday that most people cannot find. So consider for example the following three words: 'reading', 'service', and 'stick'. These words look ostensibly unconnected but there is a fourth word that can link all three of them. Being able to find this hidden link between them is something of a creative challenge, and is the basis of a well-known test of creativity known as the *Remote Associates Test*. So in the example here, the correct answer would be . . .

[here's the answer coming up . . .]

. . . the answer is 'lip', because reading, service, and stick are all related to lip in some way ('lip reading', 'lip service', 'lipstick'). In the Remote Associates Test every question involves a set of three words and the task is to find the hidden 'convergent' link between them. So another question is 'wise', 'work', 'tower' where the correct answer would be 'clock' ('clockwise', 'clockwork', and 'clock tower'). It takes a certain amount of creativity to bring this hidden link to the forefront of the mind, because it involves detecting associations across otherwise unrelated dimensions. So the question arises: Do synaesthetes—adept at habitually pairing dimensions in unusual ways like sounds and tastes—easily pair together other types of concept in unusual ways too? Are they more creative than the average person, even aside from synaesthesia itself? When the Remote Associates Test was carried out on a sample of synaesthetes by Jamie Ward and his colleagues, synaesthetes performed significantly better than a group of non-synaesthetes. This suggests that the synaesthetes tested in that study were particularly good at this type of creative convergent thinking. Other studies have concluded that synaesthetes also appear to have creativity imbued in their personality traits. But before I describe these findings, we need to first consider how we might take a scientific measure of someone's personality.

Do synaesthetes have creative personality traits?

Personality develops from multifaceted influences, determined by both our genes and our environment. Understanding the intricate make-up of someone's personality allows us to predict how he or she might think, feel, and act in any given situation. And at first glance it seems like personality is something we all understand well and can 'read' in our daily encounters with others. From intuition alone, we can probably say that one group of people (e.g. Americans who vote Republican) seem to have different personalities to another group of people (e.g. Americans who vote Democrat). But it is a complex thing to describe scientifically. What exactly is it that makes a Republican different to a Democrat given that we are all multifaceted and different to each other in so many ways? And if we could sum up the personality difference between Republicans and Democrats could we apply that logic to other groups? Golfers versus soccer players? Teachers versus police officers? Old versus young? Men versus women? Or might it all become too complicated?

One elegant way to measure personality is to consider it as having component parts, or *factors*. Ernest Tupes and Raymond Christal defined five factors of personality which were later refined by researchers such as Lewis Goldberg, Paul Costa, and Robert McCrae and are widely known today as: *Conscientiousness, Extraversion, Agreeableness, Neuroticism,* and *Openness to Experience.* The factor of Conscientiousness relates to the importance placed on self-discipline, organization, and duty:

someone who places great importance on these things is high in Conscientiousness. Extraversion is, as we might expect, the degree to which one is outgoing and assertive but also relates to one's sense of adventure. Agreeableness describes one's level of compassion for others, one's helpfulness, and one's degree of modesty. Neuroticism describes how much one is anxious versus emotionally stable, and one's degree of impulse-control. And importantly for us, the fifth trait is Openness to Experience, a trait reflecting not only intellectual curiosity, but also artistic interest and imagination. To some extent then, it is the trait of Openness to Experience that might be particularly high in people with a creative bent.

This model of personality, divided into key traits representing stable factors of human temperament, has been widely accepted both within and outside academic circles. These traits can be measured using simple questionnaires, with names such as the *Big Five Inventory* or *Five Factor Inventory*. Such questionnaires present a number of statements for each personality factor, for example: 'I am someone who worries a lot' and 'I am someone who can be tense' for Neuroticism; or 'I am someone who assumes the best about people' and 'I am someone who has a forgiving nature' for Agreeableness. Filling out the questionnaire involves scoring each statement from 1 to 5 to rate how much it applies to one's own personality. Scores are then aggregated within each factor to give an overall picture of one's Conscientiousness, Extraversion, Agreeableness, Neuroticism, and Openness to Experience. For example, a quick check of my own scores suggests I am about as Extraverted as the next person and pretty Agreeable, but fairly high in Neuroticism (a bit of a worrier) and extremely high in Openness to Experience (being an art-loving professor) and Contentiousness (a bit of a perfectionist). The five factors model has been validated not only cross-culturally, but also from neuroscientific studies. So the extent to which someone shows the trait of Neuroticism co-varies with the volume of the brain in a region associated with threat, punishment, and negative affect—just as one might expect from this particular personality trait. Interestingly, Openness to Experience has been the hardest factor to pin down to one region of the brain, possibly because the trait consists of several facets (e.g. intellectual curiosity, artistic interest) and so it has been linked to activity in several areas of the brain that serve a range of functions, including emotion formation, learning, and memory.

But if Openness to Experience is the personality trait reflecting artistic interest and imagination do we find this to be an elevated trait among synaesthetes? Psychologist Michael Banissy and his team tested a group of synaesthetes and found they scored significantly higher than controls on this personality trait. The same was shown in a study in the Netherlands and another in France—the latter showing not only higher Openness to Experience but also a related trait of Absorption, which reflects an individual's enjoyment of imaginative activities. Although these three studies also differed in some ways (variously disagreeing on Neuroticism, Conscientiousness, and Agreeableness) they all agreed on one finding in particular: the synaesthetes they tested were particularly high in Openness to Experience, which relates in part to artistic interest and imagination. And synaesthetes have other skills too that could help them in artistic endeavours, including a good eye and a good memory for colour. We will explore more of these abilities below.

Do synaesthetes have better perception?

Psychologists refer to human abilities under different headings and one division is between *perception* and *cognition*. The former refers to how the brain processes information from the outside world entering via sensory organs (i.e. things we hear, see, taste, etc.) and the latter refers to our ability to manipulate abstract thought (e.g. to recall things from memory, manipulate language, solve reasoning problems, and so on). In both these domains synaesthetes appear to have a number of advantages, and a small sprinkling of disadvantages. For example, in one study on perception, a group of odour-colour synaesthetes were better than a group of non-synaesthetes at discriminating between different odours, and better too at discriminating the difference between colours. Likewise, in another study, grapheme-colour synaesthetes were better than non-synaesthetes in discriminating between colours and between shapes. These test-subjects had to detect the 'odd man out' in a set of colours where differences were extremely subtle, or tell the difference between a perfect and imperfect circle. Synaesthetes did this with greater accuracy but their visual advantages came with one particular cost: although grapheme-colour synaesthetes were better at detecting colour and shape they were worse at detecting motion. In the motion test, subjects were shown a group of random dots moving on a computer screen within which a small cluster of dots were moving in the same direction. Test subjects had to detect this motion and say whether it was moving left or right. Synaesthetes performed relatively poorly in this task. Interestingly, this play off between the detection of colour/shape (performed well by synaesthetes) and motion (performed badly by synaesthetes) mirrors how colour/shape and motion interact in the brain.

All people show a competition in the brain between areas encoding motion on the one hand, and colour/shape on the other: when one area is supressed, the other performs well. For example, a study by Vincent Walsh and his colleagues used a technique called *transcranial magnetic stimulation* (or TMS) to supress the motion area of the brain in a group of average test subjects. TMS can prevent a small area of the cortex from functioning in the normal way, but only for a limited time period. When this time has passed (often just a matter of minutes) the brain functions normally again. This temporary disruption in the brain is brought about by placing a *TMS coil* near the head of the test-subject. This device generates a magnetic field producing small electric currents in the region of the brain immediately under the coil, and supresses that small brain area. When Vincent Walsh and his colleagues used TMS to supress the motion area of the brain (a region known as v5), they found the expected consequence on motion detection: test-subjects were suddenly slower to detect moving Xs on a computer screen. Unexpectedly however, the disruption of the motion centre seemed to *help* in colour/shape detection: subjects were suddenly faster at detecting a green X in an array of red Xs and green dashes. This suggests that motion competes with colour/shape in the brain. This competition could explain why a benefit for synaesthetes in the latter manifested itself alongside a corresponding deficit in the former. This conclusion also has supporting evidence in brain imaging. We saw in Chapter 2 that synaesthetes have differences in white and grey matter in some areas of the brain and, of particular relevance here, this includes region v5. Colour-synaesthetes show reduced grey matter in areas of the brain that process motion, and this may be linked to their poorer performance in motion-detecting tasks.

Do synaesthetes have better cognition?

One area where synaesthetes appear to excel is in their memory. Synaesthetes are better than non-synaesthetes at remembering colours in the environment. They also perform well when recalling words they have memorized, and perhaps also when recalling individual graphemes (i.e. letters and numbers). In one study, Bradley Gibson and his colleagues tested a group of grapheme-colour synaesthetes who had coloured letters but not numbers, and these synaesthetes were better than control subjects at recalling letters in particular. This is important because it suggests that the memory advantages for synaesthetes were restricted to graphemes that triggered colours, and this might be accounted for by *Dual-Coding Theory*. Dual-Coding relates to the tendency for stimuli to be better remembered if they are elaborated with many different details. So if I asked you to remember that I recently purchased a pen, you would probably remember this object better if you knew, too, that it was made of silver and had a black lid. These additional features (silver, black lid) make the object more robustly encoded in your memory and so easier to recall at a later date. In a similar way, synaesthetic colours perhaps provide additional memory-features for letter-colour synaesthetes when recalling lists of letters, and of course these extra features are not available to most other people.

Although a Dual-Coding Theory is a sensible explanation of Bradley Gibson's findings, it does not seem to be the whole story. Dual-Coding alone predicts that synaesthetes should have good memories only for things that have been 'elaborated' in their memories (i.e. things that trigger synaesthesia) but this does not appear to be the case. Synaesthetes also out-perform non-synaesthetes in their memory for things *unrelated* to synaesthesia such as meaningless images of *fractals* (abstract spiralling patterns). These cannot have been 'dual-coded' in memory because they do not have synaesthetic colours, so how might we explain this? Perhaps synaesthetes simply have a good ability to perceptually organize information to make retention and recall more efficient. But these advantages appear to be tied to the general *domain* of their synaesthesia, even if not limited to inducers themselves. So even though fractals do not trigger synaesthesia, they are better remembered only by synaesthetes with visual concurrents (grapheme-colour synaesthetes not synaesthetes who experience tastes). Such broad visual advantages are mirrored in visual cortex activation, which is greater for visual synaesthetes even when not experiencing synaesthesia. Simply looking at *gabor patches*, for example, which look like tightly spaced parallel bars and do not trigger synaesthesia, can cause greater activation for visual synaesthetes compared to the average person. So synaesthetes appear to have different visual organization, which is likely to be implicated in their ability to recall visual information, whether this triggers synaesthesia or not.

As well as advantages in memory there are also cognitive difficulties, at least for some synaesthetes in some cognitive tasks. One study looked at the ability to perform mental arithmetic for a group of sequence-space synaesthetes, who mentally project numbers into space. We saw examples of these types of spatial mental 'number forms' in Chapter 1 (Figure 2(b)). In 2009, a group of sequence-space synaesthetes were asked to perform a series of mental arithmetic problems that involved addition, subtraction, multiplication, and division. The aim of the study was to see whether there were advantages to being able to mentally project numbers, but the results of the study were initially surprising. Instead of having advantages, synaesthetes actually performed worse but only in multiplication—they were perfectly fine in addition, subtraction, and division. On closer inspection these results makes sense. Multiplication is different to other functions such as addition in that multiplication relies heavily on verbal memorization. Remember all those hours you spent repeating your times-tables? This helped you learn them as verbal facts—a little like remembering the words to a song. So what happened to sequence-space synaesthetes in their multiplication test? One interpretation is that they tried to rely on their spatial projection of numbers to perform the calculations. This could be a useful strategy for functions like addition, but would hold them back in the heavily verbal skill of multiplication. So having a mental projection of numbers was a disadvantage, if synaesthetes tried to rely too heavily on it where it was not appropriate for the task.

Are synaesthetes better at cross-sensory processing?

One important area to consider is whether synaesthetes perform better in cross-sensory or cross-modal processing. The former relates to combining information across the senses (e.g. integrating things we see with the sounds they make) while the latter involves combining information across any two qualities more broadly, for example relating sound to meaning (e.g. working out that a high-pitch squeak likely means a mouse is nearby rather than an elephant). Synaesthesia is a type of cross-sensory or cross-modal skill par excellence, because it unites different qualities in automatic and exceptional ways. It has been said that cross-modality or cross-sensory integration might therefore be more deeply ingrained in synaesthetes. So are they better than the average person at uniting what they hear with what they see in the world around them, or uniting sounds with meaning? Even aside from synaesthesia itself? The results in this field of research are somewhat conflicting: some studies suggest synaesthetes perform better than the average person in such tasks, while other studies show synaesthetes perform no better, or even worse.

Evidence of advantages for synaesthetes in cross-modal processing comes from a study I ran with Kaitlyn Bankieris looking at the sounds of words. To understand this study we have to first understand the link between sound and meaning in languages across the world. In the English language for example, it is mostly the case that the sounds of words do not relate directly to their meanings. We cannot guess what a word means simply from how it sounds, so there is nothing cat-like for example about the sounds 'C' and 'A' and 'T'. Instead we have to learn the meaning of 'cat' explicitly. So although a few words in English do give clues to their meaning (e.g. onomatopoeia such as 'hiss') there is generally very little 'sound symbolism' in the words we use. But other languages of the world do contain words with sound symbolism. As a result, we can guess their meanings even if we are a non-speaker. Ask yourself whether the word 'hui' in Chinese means light or dark? Does the word 'nana' in Gujarati mean small or big? Does the word 'ma' in Korean mean up or down? If you guessed light, small, and up (as people tend to do at above-chance levels) then you have correctly detected their sound symbolism: the subtle and almost mysterious quality of certain words that allows us to correctly guess what they mean. Sound symbolism is a type of *cross-modal* association (i.e. it links the modalities of sound and word-meaning) so is reminiscent of synaesthesia (e.g. linking modalities such as colour and word meaning). So are synaesthetes particularly good at sound symbolism games? We found that they were.

In our study we gave a group of synaesthetes 400 foreign words from a hundred different languages (Albanian, Gujarati, Indonesian, Korean, etc.) and asked them to guess the meaning of each word. We did the same with a group of non-synaesthete control subjects and in each case we gave two possible meanings (e.g. does 'hui' mean light or dark?) so that a pure guess rate would be 50 per cent accurate. We found—as expected—that the non-synaesthete control group, like all average people, performed better than chance. They were correct about 55 per cent of the time, and wrong only 45 per cent. Synaesthetes however were even better: their accuracy was almost 60 per cent and this was statistically better than the average person. A similar finding was produced by Simon Lacey and Kelly McCormick, at Emory University. They showed that synaesthetes have stronger intuitive links for sound symbolism even for nonsense words. In their study, synaesthetes and non-synaesthetes saw geometric shapes which were rounded or jagged, and they heard the nonsense words 'lomo' and 'kekay'. These particular nonsense words carry a sound symbolism for all people: linguists such as Alan Nielsen have shown that words containing *liquid consonants* like L tend to be intuitively associated to rounded shapes, while words containing *stop consonants* such as K tend to be intuitively associated to jagged shapes. Lacey and McCormick showed that synaesthetes had more automatic and instinctive cross-modal associations between 'lomo' and rounded shapes, and between 'kekay' and jagged shapes, compared to the average person. So what can we conclude from this? Perhaps synaesthetes are powerhouses of cross-modality who excel in all types of cross-modal ability. But unfortunately, the picture becomes less clear when other findings are taken into account.

Although synaesthetes excelled at linguistic cross-modality, they were less exceptional in other cross-modal—particularly cross-sensory—tasks. For example, Lacey and McCormick also tested whether synaesthetes were different than average people when linking across the senses of sight and sound. Their study was based on an intuitive association between sound and vision we all share, which is that sounds high in pitch are intuitively felt to be small or elevated in space. We will speak more about this in Chapter 5, but I point out for now that while synaesthetes had stronger intuitions about sound symbolism in language, they were no different than non-synaesthetes in the strength of their cross-sensory correspondences between sound and vision.

At least three further studies also looked at cross-sensory integration in synaesthetes but their results were conflicting. These studies examined a cross-sensory artefact we are all susceptible to, known as the *Sound Induced Flash Illusion*. The illusion is produced when sounds (e.g. beeps) occur together with flashes of light; the sound influences how many light flashes we think we see. Two beeps and one flash is often mistakenly perceived as two flashes. The effect is quite remarkable, and arises from our having assimilated together the cross-sensory information from vision and audition. Now, if synaesthetes are particularly strong cross-sensory assimilators, perhaps they might be especially susceptible to this illusion. Unfortunately, the science is inconclusive: one study showed synaesthetes were more susceptible, another showed they were less susceptible, and a third showed they were just the same as non-synaesthetes. However, the factor of age might play a role here. In recent studies led by Alberta Ipser in my own lab and Beat Meier in Switzerland, we have found that synaesthesia appears to decline in older people, and this should mean older synaesthetes experience the Sound Induced Flash Illusion less than younger ones. (This is because losing synaesthesia means losing cross-sensory sensitivities, which means losing the illusion.) And this seems to fit with all three studies: where synaesthetes showed the illusion, they were younger than when they did not. In summary, although synaesthetes showed strong cross-modality differences in language, there is less evidence for differences in cross-*sensory* tasks, although the effects here may be moderated by age.

Is synaesthesia a factor in health and mental well-being?

To end this chapter we turn to the question of health and well-being, and start by asking whether synaesthetic sensations are pleasant or troubling. In most cases, adults with synaesthesia have had synaesthesia since childhood and would say it is not obtrusive, it does not affect day-to-day life in any negative way, and it feels perfectly normal to experience the world in this way. But individual people react differently to having synaesthesia. Some feel indifferent, some feel highly positive (and I cannot stress this enough), while some experience difficulties. In this final camp, there are several forms of synaesthesia that can actually cause pain. Some synaesthetes have reported that thinking very hard about colours in synaesthesia can cause flashes of headache. In rare cases, synaesthesia can cause pain directly, as in *mirror-touch synaesthesia* in which synaesthetes can experience touch or sometimes pain when they see other people hurt (see Figure 10 and Box 5).

Of course the vast majority of synaesthesias do *not* cause pain but some forms can nonetheless be overwhelming if they involve strong or unpleasant sensations. People with lexical-gustatory synaesthesia for example (who taste words) can experience intrusive or unpleasant flavours in the mouth. Words can sometimes trigger the taste of vomit, ear-wax, mucous, and so on. On the other hand, they can also trigger the taste of chocolate or the taste of melted cheese, both very pleasant in their own right but not necessarily pleasant together when triggered by neighbouring words in the same sentence. Perhaps one way to understand this better is to turn to James Wannerton, the President of the UK Synaesthesia Association. James recently produced a synaesthetic map of the London Underground tube (train) system (see Figure 11) which replaces station names with the tastes he experiences when he passes through each station and reads its

Box 5

Figure 10 shows a procedure used by Medina and DePasquale (2017) to study mirror-touch synaesthesia. Mirror-touch synaesthetes feel touch on their own body when they see someone else being touched. In some cases, this can even cause pain if the observed touch caused pain to the person actually being touched. Brain imaging shows unusual activation in the somatosensory cortex of mirror-touch synaesthetes. Somatosensory regions in the parietal lobe play a key role in the feeling of touch for all people and can also activate when observing others being touched. Mirror-touch synaesthetes show significantly more activation than control subjects

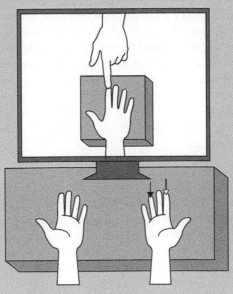

10. Experimental set up to study mirror-touch synaesthesia.

(continued)

Box 5 Continued

suggesting mirror-touch synaesthesia may be caused by an over-active mirror-touch system. Using the procedure here, Medina and DePasquale tested forty-five mirror-touch synaesthetes and showed their synaesthetic touch sensations were dependent on body position. Here, the synaesthete watches a video of a right hand, palm down, being touched at the tip of its index finger. The two hands at the bottom are the synaesthete's own, and the white arrow points to her corresponding fingertip (right index finger). Because the synaesthete's hands are palm up they do not match the posture on-screen. This mismatch lessened the synaesthetic touch sensations; these tended to occur more often when video hand and synaesthete's hand matched (palm up or palm down). Mismatched posture also affected the synaesthetic touch's location (e.g. viewed touch on the fingertip pad, palms up, was felt as synaesthetic touch on the back of the synaesthete's fingertip when palm down). In some cases, the synaesthetic touch was felt on a different finger, for example, shown by the black arrow. This is a specular (i.e. mirror) version of where video touch occurred, being two digits in from the left. Overall results suggest that synaesthetes' body schemas influence synaesthetic touch.

name. When travelling a few minutes on the District and Circle Line, James Wannerton tastes candle wax followed by chewing gum, two types of chocolate mints then tomato soup, spam, fruit cake, and mucous. Travelling on the Central Line he tastes bacon followed by Yorkshire pudding then aerosol spray, while on the Bakerloo Line, he tastes pie crust followed by vinegar. Some tastes are unpleasant by their nature and some unpleasant by their juxtaposition. So although synaesthesia is a heterogeneous, multifaceted condition with many pleasant sensations, it has the

11. Photograph of graphic artwork *Tastes of London* 1964–2013 by James Wannerton.

possibility of unpleasant sensations from time to time, or from one synaesthesia type to another.

Even if the synaesthesia is itself pleasant, there are other difficulties it might bring. Between 2014 and 2018 we ran a large study at the universities of Edinburgh and Sussex to screen many thousands of people for grapheme-colour synaesthesia. And as well as screening for synaesthesia, we took a detailed health history from every test-subject. Their health histories revealed that people with grapheme-colour synaesthesia were significantly more likely than the average person to be diagnosed with anxiety disorder. We verified our finding by repeating the study a second time on a new and larger sample, and found the results confirmed: rates of anxiety disorder were higher in synaesthetes. As I write this book these findings are still rather new and their explanation is not yet clear. In Chapter 2 we saw that at least one research lab has speculated that synaesthesia may be caused by mutations in serotonin pathways genes, given that synaesthesia-like sensations can be induced from drugs which act on serotonin pathways such as LSD. (Remember that serotonin is a neurotransmitter which plays a role in relaying signals from one part of the brain to another.) Anxiety disorder, too, has been linked to serotonin receptors, giving a second reason to further investigate these pathways in synaesthetes. But in truth, we really have absolutely no understanding of serotonin in synaesthesia so it would be premature to draw any definitive conclusions about its potential role for synaesthetes with anxiety disorder. Our study simply provides evidence that there may be repercussions in the mental health of grapheme-colour synaesthetes, leading to higher rates of anxiety for some synaesthetes.

Anxiety disorder may not be the only challenging experience faced by some people with synaesthesia. A study by Manchester researcher Helen Carruthers and colleagues screened for grapheme-colour synaesthesia within a large sample of patients with IBS (irritable bowel syndrome). IBS is characterized by visceral hypersensitivity but IBS patients also happen to show sensitivity to external stimuli like sound. Carruthers and colleagues also found higher than expected rates of synaesthesia in IBS patients compared with a control sample. However, our own recent health-screening study has failed to replicate this finding, in that self-reported diagnoses of IBS were no higher in our synaesthetes than controls. Despite this ambivalence over the visceral sensitivities of IBS, there is evidence for *other* types of sensitivities in synaesthetes. Recent studies show that people with grapheme-colour synaesthesia can experience uncomfortable sensory sensitivities. One way to test for visual sensitivities is to present *visual gratings*—parallel black and white lines. Depending on the thickness of the lines, gratings are sometimes unpleasant to look at, and can cause visual experiences such as shimmers or even discomfort. And these sensitivities are especially strong in grapheme-colour synaesthetes. Finally, when describing their sensory sensitivities in a questionnaire, synaesthetes reported more-than-average sensory overload from everyday sights, sounds, odours, and so on. Conversely though, synaesthetes may also be *hypo*-sensitive, in that they can sometimes feel *under*-stimulated and so actively go out of their way to seek certain odours, tastes, textures, etc. It is curious to note that sensory sensitivities are also a quality of another well-known and well-studied phenomenon: autism spectrum conditions. Indeed, there is more than a passing similarity between synaesthesia and autism, which we will cover briefly now.

In 2018 we administered a standard questionnaire known as the *Autism Spectrum Quotient* to people with synaesthesia and to people with autism. This questionnaire has five sections, four relating to autistic-like traits of impairment (in social skills, communication, imagination, and attention-switching) and one relating to autistic-like advantages (in attention-to-detail). We found that synaesthetes had autistic-like traits linked to enhanced attention-to-detail, but in the absence of the traditional impairments that otherwise define autism. But two seminal studies in 2013 by Janina Neufeld and Simon Baron-Cohen showed that grapheme-colour synaesthesia was more common in people with Asperger's syndrome (high functioning autism) compared to the general population. This finding does not mean that people with synaesthesia are likely to also have autism; the overwhelming majority of people with synaesthesia do not. It simply means that people with autism had more synaesthesia than we would otherwise expect. And in cases where people are diagnosed with both conditions, something quite remarkable happens. Post-doctoral researcher James Hughes ran a study in my lab showing that having both synaesthesia and autism gives a high likelihood that the individual will develop some type of remarkable talent.

Talent is known to occur in a surprising number of people with autism, and when this arises it is referred to as *savant syndrome*.

Autistic people with savant syndrome can have exceptional skills such as the ability to memorize thousands of digits, or to perform amazing feats of mental calculation (e.g. multiplying two six-digit numbers almost instantaneously), or they have unusual skills like calendar-counting (i.e. knowing the day of the week for any date in history) or the ability draw complex scenes in photographic detail (e.g. drawing highly detailed aerial views of the city of London after just one fly-over) and so on. What makes these skills 'savant' in nature is when they co-occur with developmental deficits such as autism. Darold Treffert, perhaps the world's leading expert in savant syndrome, describes savant skills as 'islands of genius' within a landscape of disability. Our research has suggested a fascinating link between these 'islands of genius' and having synaesthesia.

In one recent study we tested three groups of people: people with autism who have an exceptional talent (i.e. savants), people with autism but no exceptional talent, and neurotypical controls (i.e. not savants, not autistic). We screened every person for synaesthesia and found that—as expected—synaesthesia was more common in people with autism. But when we broke down the autistic individuals into their two groups—savants and non-savants—we found that rates of synaesthesia were high only in the former. So having synaesthesia was somehow tied to having an exceptional skill in people with autism. We have understood this link in the following way. Remember first that people with synaesthesia have slight added abilities whether they are savants or not. Above we saw they have slightly better colour perception, memory, language abilities, and a host of other small advantages. But when those advantages are coupled with autism, something exceptional appears to happen. We believe this may be because autism gives several other skills which can hone the talents of synaesthesia into *exceptional* talents. For example, people with autism sometimes have obsessive traits which might give them obsessive urges to rehearse. If they over-rehearse their talents from synaesthesia, these could potentially develop into the extraordinary talents of savant syndrome.

Links between synaesthesia and savant abilities have also been described in detail by writer Daniel Tammet a well-known savant and synaesthete. Among Daniel's remarkable savant talents is the ability to recall from memory 22,514 digits of the mathematical constant pi (π) and Daniel has provided eloquent insight into how his (grapheme-colour and sequence-personality) synaesthesia helps him achieves such remarkable feats. In his book *Born on a Blue Day* Daniel explains:

> Numbers are my friends and they are always around me. Each one is unique and has its own personality. Eleven is friendly and five is loud... Some are big—23, 667, 1,179—while others are small: 6,13,581. Some are beautiful, like 333, and some are ugly, like 289. To me, every number is special... The number one, for example, is a brilliant and bright white... Thirty-seven is lumpy like porridge... Using my own synaesthetic experiences since early childhood, I have grown up with the ability to handle and calculate huge numbers in my head without any conscious effort... When I look at a sequence of numbers, my head begins to fill with colours, shapes and textures that knit together spontaneously to form a visual landscape... To recall each digit, I simply retrace the different shapes and textures in my head and read the numbers out of them... As the sequence of digits grows, my numerical landscapes become more complex and layered, until—as with pi—they are like an entire country in my mind, composed of numbers. This is how I 'see' the first twenty digits of pi [see Figure 12].

Throughout this chapter we have seen that synaesthetes are different from the average person in a number of ways, which go beyond the fact that they have coloured letters, tasty words, time in space, or other synaesthetic sensations. Synaesthesia appears to come with a number of benefits making it a 'gift' for many

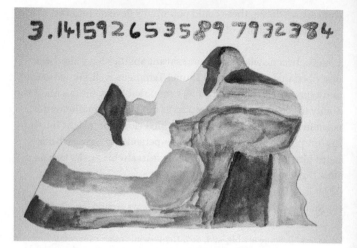

12. Daniel Tammet's synaesthetic number landscape for the first twenty digits of the mathematical constant π.

synaesthetes. The remarkable descriptions of someone like Daniel Tammet show how synaesthesia can operate in individuals with great talent for example. But synaesthesia can also bring challenges, making it akin to a 'condition' for other synaesthetes. Together these advantages and disadvantages make up a very particular psychological profile. But when do these differences start to emerge, and where does synaesthesia itself come from? In Chapter 5 we will examine the roots of synaesthesia, looking along the way at the effects of nature and nurture. We will find a fascinating picture of how biology and environment conspire together to bring about the richly embroidered world of the synaesthete.

Chapter 5
Where does synaesthesia come from? The role of genetics and learning

In Chapter 2 we looked into the brains of synaesthetes and saw that synaesthesia is likely caused by some type of *cross-communication* that allows one cortical area (e.g. a colour region) to fire in response to incoming signals at a different cortical area (e.g. a region recognizing letters). But why are the brains of synaesthetes so 'communicative' and how exactly do synaesthetic sensations form? In this chapter we will ask whether synaesthesia is predetermined in the genes, or based on learning from the environment. We will see that both these things are true: there are strong genetic indicators in the DNA (deoxyribonucleic acid) of synaesthetes, but the *type* of sensations they develop (e.g. green 7s, red As) can be influenced by what they learn after they are born. By considering how different features become paired up in the minds of synaesthetes, we can start to understand where these associations come from. So let us start by first looking more closely at synaesthetic associations themselves.

Where do synesthetic pairings come from? Similarities among synaesthetes

Why might the letter A be red for one particular synaesthete, and not yellow, green, orange, or another colour altogether? In scientific parlance we might ask why certain *inducers* come to be paired with certain synaesthetic *concurrents*? In recent years, scientists have come to realize that the mapping between elements in synaesthesia (between an A and the colour red, say) is not completely chaotic and random, but to some extent logical and regulated. You may be surprised to learn that synaesthetes follow a set of unconscious 'rules' when they pair together letters with colours, or words with flavours, and so on. And most surprising of all, even non-synaesthetes have synaesthesia-like associations which bear a striking resemblance to genuine synaesthesia. It may be precisely for this reason that audiences find synaesthetes' experiences so enjoyable as art forms (as we saw in Chapter 3). So let us explore this further.

Until around twenty years ago scientists believed that synaesthetic pairings—such as a certain letter paired with a certain colour—were completely random and idiosyncratic from one synaesthete to the next. Scientists had not yet been able to harness the power of the internet to recruit large numbers of synaesthetes, and so were forced to study just a handful of synaesthetes at any one time; this tends to exaggerate their differences. Two synaesthetes will often disagree and I have heard as much from members of my own household: one says Tuesday is orange while another says it is Christmas green, and yet another says it is tweed-coloured grey. But as soon as the internet allowed scientists to recruit large groups of synaesthetes, surprising patterns emerged. Two studies in 2005, from my own lab and from a team in Australia led by Anina Rich, looked at several hundred synaesthetes for the very first time. When we compared their colours for letters, we did not find the chaotic idiosyncrasies we might have expected, but clear patterns across the group as a whole. The letter A tended to be red significantly more often than chance would predict; B tended to be blue; C tended to be yellow; and so on. So although any colours were possible, each letter had its *preferred* colour (or sometimes two colours) which allowed us to draw up a 'prototypical synaesthetic alphabet' showing the most statistically likely synaesthetic colours for each letter (see Figure 13; within

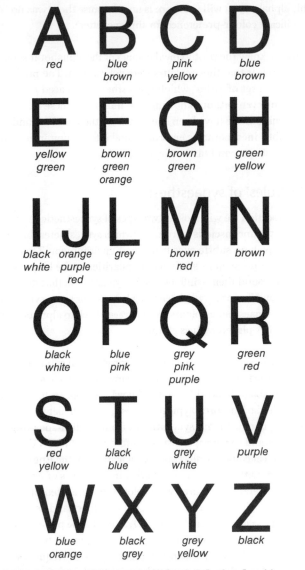

13. A representation of the prototypical synaesthetic colour(s) for letters, from a large group of grapheme-colour synaesthetes.

this alphabet you will see there is no K because there was no significant colour-preference for this one letter).

Once we knew the prototypical colours of the alphabet it soon became clear that these colours were not random. The preferences followed a set of 'rules', which synaesthetes appeared to be following even without knowing it. A number of these rules show that synaesthetes have been learning from the world around them and subtly incorporating environmental information into their colours, shapes, and tastes of synaesthesia.

The 'rules' of synaesthesia

In this section we will look at two types of synaesthetic learning. The first is unconscious learning in which synaesthetes, like all people, pick up subtle cues from their environment. This information—such as statistical regularities in the languages spoken around them—influences the synaesthesia that develops. The second is more *explicit* learning because for some synaesthetes at least, synaesthetic colours can be traced back to alphabet books or toys they played with as children.

Unconscious learning comes from environmental submersion; simply growing up in a particular environment teaches us all sorts of things about the world. And this knowledge appears to influence synaesthesia. The 'prototypical' synaesthetic alphabet in Figure 13 happens to come from synaesthetes from English-speaking countries and so perhaps unsurprisingly we have found that their prototypical colours reflect statistical features of the English language. Letters that are used *often* in the words of English (e.g. A, S) tend to be paired with colours that are often talked about in English (e.g. red, yellow). On the other hand, letters that are used *less often* in English (e.g. Q, J) tend to be paired with colours that are talked about *less* often (e.g. purple, turquoise). Here we use the term 'linguistic frequency': high-frequency (commonly used) letters tend to be paired with high frequency colour words. This influence of frequency is no surprise because human beings happen to be particularly good frequency counters. We have instinctive knowledge of all kinds of frequency statistics, so know intuitively what we encounter often (e.g. jeans, t-shirts, rings) and what we encounter less often (e.g. cravats, bow-ties, brooches). And frequency knowledge is put to work in synaesthesia—albeit unconsciously. Most synaesthetes do not know and cannot state that they have a frequency rule colouring their letters. Researcher Gian Beeli, Daniel Smilek, and colleagues have shown that frequency is also tied to the brightness and saturation of synaesthetic colours, because even the specific *shades* of colour taken by common letters tend to be lighter and richer than shades taken by uncommon letters. And other types of environmental linguistic knowledge is also subconsciously evaluated, such as the *ordering* of letters: research has shown that the first letter in alphabets around the world is synaesthetically more distinct in colour than the rest of the alphabet.

So synaesthetes absorb information from their environment and unconsciously apply this to their synaesthesia. And not just in colours. In earlier chapters, we introduced sequence-personality synaesthesia, which imbues sequences such as letters with specific personas. For example, letter A might be a motherly female, B might be a mischievous toddler, C a sinister young man, and so on. These synaesthetic personalities also appear to be influenced by environment because they tend to reflect the society that is contemporary to the synaesthete. We are lucky enough to have reports of sequence-personality synaesthesia from the 19th century, and these older reports mention personas that are society girls and housekeepers, while modern accounts describe contemporary archetypes such as 'frat boys' and 'goths' (i.e. members of college fraternities and enthusiasts of Gothic rock music, respectively). All this suggests that synaesthetic personalities, too, are moulded around lifetime experiences. Consider, too, touch-colour synaesthetes, who sense colours when they touch objects with their fingers. In some cases these phantom colours share qualities found in the real world. For example, one physical quality of smooth objects is that they are bright and shiny because they reflect light more than rough objects. So it is interesting to note that synaesthetes' colours when touching smooth objects tend to be lighter than when touching rough objects (at least for the small number of touch-colour synaesthetes we have studied so far).

And synaesthetic tastes, too, are influenced by what lexical-gustatory (word-taste) synaesthetes have eaten growing up. Foods that the synaesthete ate most often as a child are statistically most likely to arise as synaesthetic tastes in adulthood—meaning that lexical-gustatory synaesthesia often has a 'childlike' quality (e.g. heavy on the chocolate and light on alcohol). And tastes do not spring up from words randomly, but through learning the network of sounds and meanings in the synaesthete's native language. In a series of studies conducted with colleagues Sarah Haywood and Jamie Ward, I have found that the first tastes to emerge are likely to be logical associations between food words and their flavours. For example, the word 'peach' starts to taste of peaches. But as the synaesthetic child learns more words, these tastes spread through his or her vocabulary via the sounds of words. Suddenly, any word that shares speech sounds with 'peach'—like 'beach' or 'reach' or 'cheap' or 'chimneysweep'—might suddenly start to taste of peaches too. And the taste itself might morph and develop from peaches, to peach yoghurt, to peach hair conditioner, and so on. All this means that a seemingly chaotic adult system can nonetheless be traced back to the synaesthete's childhood diet, and to his or her exposure to language.

Let us end by considering a more explicit type of learning. At least some grapheme-colour synaesthetes are influenced by early ABC books or alphabet toys, whose colours appear to become imprinted onto their lifelong synaesthesia. This happens relatively rarely—in only 6 per cent of cases studied by Nathan Witthoft, and as few as one in 150 cases studied by Anina Rich. However, alphabet books can also have another type of influence on grapheme-colour synaesthetes. My own study with Jennifer Mankin suggests that synaesthetic colours can also derive from literacy mnemonics such as 'A is for apple...D is for dog...'. We asked a large numbers of people from the general population to complete phrases of the type 'A is for...' (e.g. A is for apple). A second group of people were asked for the most common colours of these objects (e.g. apples tend to be red). We found that these colours statistically predict the colourful alphabets of synaesthetes. In other words, A tends to be prototypically red for synaesthetes perhaps because A is for apple and apples are prototypically red. This relationship is an underlying trend that can be seen across large groups of synaesthetes, even if it is not apparent in every synaesthete on a case-by-case basis.

What we appear to be seeing is that synaesthesia reflects our environment, and perhaps especially our environment during childhood. And synaesthesia certainly does 'grow' over time along with the growing child. Between 2005 and 2009, I followed a group of children with grapheme-colour synaesthesia as they grew older. When they were 6 years old, only one-third of their alphabets had consistent synaesthetic colours. The remaining letters fluctuated in colour from moment to moment. When we returned to test them at age 7, around half their alphabet now had fixed colours. Finally, when we returned again at age 10, around 70 per cent of their alphabets had fixed colours. All this shows that stable synaesthetic colours for individual letters emerge slowly during childhood, but their origins can be seen in children as young as 6, and perhaps even earlier. It is possible that even very young grapheme-colour synaesthetes have colours for shapes, even before these becomes imprinted on letters. We can infer this because researchers such as David Brang and David Eagleman have shown letters with similar shapes like 'd' and 'b' are likely to be more similar in their synaesthetic colours than letters that look different such as 'd' and 'j'. Combined with what we have learned above, it seems that synaesthetic colours for letters depend not only on literacy acquisition (i.e. learning that 'A is for apple') but earlier stages in development, beginning perhaps as colourful associations for squares, circles, and other geometric shapes.

In this section, I have shown that synaesthesia is not random or chaotic, but rule-based and coherent, although more accurately, it is probably somewhere in-between. Although scientists are able to detect some regularities in the associations of synaesthetes, and although these are sometimes rule-based, these rules can be well-hidden and are often *trends* rather than absolutes. So although A tends to be red more than any other colour, it is only red for about 40 per cent of synaesthetes. For the rest it can have any colour at all, and different colours from synaesthete to synaesthete. And it is this variation that made early scientists see idiosyncrasies rather than coherence, chaos rather than harmony. But the fact that red As are found around four times more often than we would predict from chance alone, or that tasty words have a complex basis linking speech sounds and flavours, is what gives the system of synaesthesia an elegant underlying structure that is hard to not appreciate.

Cross-modal correspondences in non-synaesthetes

One interesting consequence of discovering that synaesthetes follow 'rules' when mapping across the senses is the finding that non-synaesthetes do the same. Non-synaesthetes, too, pair specific qualities of sound and colour, taste and shape, colour and texture, and so on. And their rules are sometimes the same as those of synaesthetes. These synaesthesia-like associations in non-synaesthetes are called *cross-modal correspondences*, and are intuitive feelings or preferences about how the senses 'fit' together. For example, we will see below that all people have surprising preferences for the colours of sounds even if we are non-synaesthetes. Unlike true synaesthesia, these correspondences are not often felt at a conscious level, and have no veridical quality at all. They differ from true synaesthesia in their immediacy and vividness, but can nonetheless share similar mapping rules as those found in true synaesthetes.

Consider then your own intuitive associations between sound and colour. Synaesthetes with coloured music tend to follow a specific rule: their synaesthetic colours from musical notes tend to be lighter when the pitch of the note is higher. But this association also feels intuitively right for *all people* because even *non*-synaesthetes associate colours to music, using the same unconscious bias. To be convinced of this, simply imagine you are standing in front of a piano and gently tinkling the high notes, and then crashing down on the low notes. If I asked you which sound was pale yellow and which was dark purple you would likely have at least some intuition that the tinkling high notes were perhaps the pale colour while the low notes were the dark colour. And this is the same rule we find in synaesthesia: a higher pitch triggers lighter colours. This mirroring between synaesthetes and non-synaesthetes has been shown in other forms of synaesthesia too. Non-synaesthetes pairing colours to letters show greater-than-chance similarity to grapheme-colour synaesthetes. For example, both groups have a preference for A to be red. Psychologists Roi Cohen-Kadosh and Avishai Henik have also pointed out similarities between synaesthetes and non-synaesthetes in their intuitions for numbers and space. Around 60 per cent of English-speaking sequence-space synaesthetes map smaller numbers on the left side of space but larger numbers to the right, and this intuition is also felt in around 60 per cent of English non-synaesthetes too.

Sometimes cross-modal correspondences in the general population are so far buried we can barely verbalize them. I ran a study with Vera Ludwig in Edinburgh where we asked over 200 people from the general population to feel some hidden objects, and to pick a colour association for each object they felt (see Box 6 and Figure 14). For example, among the objects were a set of six

Box 6

Figure 14 shows a procedure used by Ludwig and Simner (2013) to detect implicit associations across the senses in all people. We tested 210 participants between the ages of 5 and 74 years to show that all people have systematic unconscious pairings between touch and colour. The left image shows a participant seated in front of a screen, who chooses colours from an on-screen colour palette to match by intuition the tactile qualities of objects felt one by one through the screen. Right images show the eighteen objects and their tactile qualities: six objects were flat surfaces running from smooth to rough (quantified by abrasive grit-size following the International Organization for Standardization—ISO); six objects were foam cubes running from soft to hard (quantified by a foam compression metric in Newtons per metre squared—N/m^2) and six objects were wooden blocks running from pointed to round (according to equations described fully in the original article). Although participants thought they were choosing colours randomly, the colours they chose were systematically lighter for the smoother, softer, and rounder objects. Smoother and softer objects were also matched with colours that were more saturated than when objects were rougher and harder.

flat surfaces that ranged from rough to smooth: one surface was very smooth, one was very rough, and four were increments in-between. Our test-subjects had no idea why we were asking them to pick colours and protested that their colour choices were completely random. But when we looked at the data we found a highly significant, almost perfectly linear relationship, where colours became lighter and more saturated as the objects became smoother. So although non-synaesthetes had no awareness of their texture-colour preferences, they followed this rule in our study. And of course most remarkable of all, this same

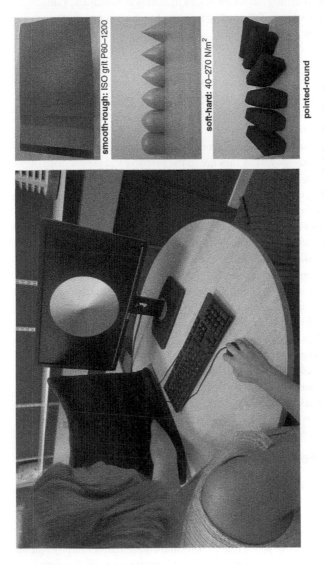

smooth-rough: ISO grit P60–1200

soft-hard: 40–270 N/m²

pointed-round

14. Experimental set-up to study cross-modal correspondence between touch and vision. See Box 6.

rule matching smoothness and lightness is exactly the rule unconsciously followed by true touch-colour synaesthetes, as we saw above.

The test-subjects in our touch-colour study ranged from 5 to 74 years of age, and correspondences between touch and colour were found even in the very youngest children. A study by psychologists Daphne Maurer and Ferrine Spector showed that children as young as 3 also have shared preference for the colours of letters: O and X were consistently coloured white and black respectively, just as they are in the prototypical associations of adult synaesthetes. And the fact that very young children had colour correspondences for letters before they had even learned the alphabet suggests they were mapping colours to basic geometric shapes (circle = white; cross = black). Psychologist Peter Walker and colleagues at Lancaster University have shown that even 3–4-month-old babies experience cross-sensory correspondences between sound and vision. Their babies watched a video of either a bouncing ball or a shape constantly morphing between spikey and rounded. While the ball was moving or the shape was morphing, the babies heard a whistle gliding from low to high pitch, and back again. Remarkably, babies had a particular preference: they looked longer at balls moving upwards to increasing pitch, and at shapes becoming spikier. This provides evidence that even very young babies have cross-sensory correspondences, which are therefore unlikely to be influenced by learning and may even be innate.

Synaesthesia in the genes

In Chapter 2 we saw that the brains of synaesthetes are structurally and/or functionally different to the average person, and a parallel science is working towards understanding whether these differences could be caused by differences in synaesthetes' genes. Genes play a role in determining all manner of physical and psychological characteristics, so it important to ask if genetics could play a role in determining the psychological traits of synaesthesia. A number of studies suggest this is almost certain to be the case. But to understand this science we first need to have a notional understanding of terms like 'genes', 'DNA', 'chromosomes', and 'the human genome' as well as how these relate to the 'exome', 'nucleotides', 'bases', and 'proteins'.

The bodily tissue of all living organisms is composed of cells, and inside each cell is a liquid called cytoplasm. Floating in the cytoplasm is the cell's nucleus which contains most of the genetic material in the form of *chromosomes*. Each chromosome (there are forty-six in most cells) is made up of a DNA molecule wrapped around a spool-like structure of proteins. This keeps the long DNA molecule wound up as a single chromosome unit. The string-like DNA molecule is often called the 'blueprint for life' because DNA carries the information that determines our characteristics: it contains the recipes for how our tissues are formed, and gives rise to what we look like, how we think, and other characteristics that make us the same or different to everyone else. So each chromosome is made of a DNA molecule, and genes themselves are just shorter stretches of that DNA within the chromosome. Although there are around 21,000 genes in the human *genome* (i.e. the sum total of all genetic information of a person), individual genes make up only about 2 per cent of our total DNA. But this 2 per cent is vital to everything we are.

Since genes and chromosomes are just stretches of DNA, they are both made of the same thing, which we can understand by looking more closely at DNA itself. We said that DNA is a string-like molecule, but it is more like a long ladder twisted into a corkscrew, and we call this shape a *double helix* (see Figure 15). The sections of this ladder are made up of chemicals called *nucleotides*. Each nucleotide contains a molecule with a substance called a *nitrogenous base*. There are four types of base, named A, C, G, or T—adenine, cytosine, guanine, and thymine—and these will be important when it comes to talking about what makes people the

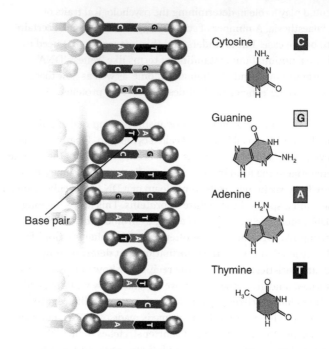

Cytosine **C**

Guanine **G**

Adenine **A**

Thymine **T**

15. The 3D structure of DNA showing nitrogenous bases: A, C, G, or T—adenine, cytosine, guanine, and thymine—and their molecular forms.

same or different from each other. Each 'rung' of the DNA ladder is made of a pair of these nucleotide base-letters, making DNA a long sequence of different As, Cs, Gs, and Ts on each side of the ladder. You can see this in Figure 15. These base-letters spell out what we call the *genetic code*. So when we talk about attempts to *sequence* the genetic code, we mean working out the order of base-letters in the DNA, running up one side of the ladder or the other.

Since each gene is just one particular stretch of DNA, genes too are composed of a long sequences of these paired base-letters.

The power in genetics comes down to the fact that our own genes carry the recipes for particular characteristics or cell behaviours. The base-letters on a gene are 'read off' by a structure called *ribosome* which uses them like a recipe to make different types of proteins. And these proteins go on to perform different functions in the human body, making us who and what we are. Here's one example: the base-letters that make up a gene called MC1R provide the ribosome ('recipe-reader') with instructions for how to make a protein that plays a role in determining—among other things—your hair colour. We might ask therefore whether synaesthesia, too, can be traced back to a certain gene or genes. To find this out we would have to locate the 'synaesthesia gene(s)' from somewhere in the human genome and this amounts to a search of over three billion base-letters.

Although the search for the synaesthesia gene(s) is still at a relatively early stage, several teams of geneticists have already taken on this challenge. My own lab is involved in one such study, headed by Simon Fisher of the Max Planck Institute in Nijmegen in the Netherlands. Our aim is to inspect the genomes of over 1,000 synaesthetes in a genome-wide association study (GWAS). The GWAS technique focusses on comparing synaesthetes to non-synaesthetes at numerous points in the genome, and these points are known as SNPs or *single nucleotide polymorphisms*. From human to human we share over 99 per cent of our DNA but what makes us individual (in height, temperament, and so on) is the 1 per cent where our DNA differs. These points of difference, or SNPs, relate to variations between people at one point in their DNA where a nucleotide's base (A, C, G, or T) is substituted for another. For example, on a particular stretch of DNA one person might have a G while another might have a T. There are around ten million SNPs in the human genome, some of which appear to have no effect at all on people. But other SNPs cause differences from person to person. For example, the trait of colour blindness is thought to be caused by this type of difference, within genes that code the proteins for colour-detecting cells in the eye.

The approach in our GWAS study of synaesthesia is to compare a group of people with synaesthesia to a group of people without, by checking SNPs in the genome to see which are associated with having synaesthesia. You might wonder why we look at the SNPs only; why not just map each person's entire genome? Simply put it is a question of money. It is still expensive to sequence and compare the entire DNA of individuals, but we can compare SNPs relatively cheaply. In the case of our GWAS study, the greatest difficulty comes in finding enough synaesthetes, because we need at least 1,000 of them—and ideally many more—but finding this number is hugely challenging given that synaesthesia is so rare. The variant we are testing, coloured letters and numbers, is found in only 1 to 2 per cent of the population, and so finding even 1,000 synaesthetes willing to give us their DNA requires sifting through at least 50,000 to 100,000 people—just for starters.

But evidence to tie synaesthesia into the person's DNA has already been provided by two key studies using a method known as *family-linkage* genetics. By looking throughout families, these seminal studies have identified chromosome 'hot spots' where genes for synaesthesia are likely to be found. Julian Asher—himself a sound-colour synaesthete, and someone we met in Chapter 1—was the first geneticist to lead a team with this goal in mind. They recruited forty-three families of synaesthetes. Each family contained more than one synaesthete, giving 121 people with synaesthesia in total, and 196 family members in the study overall. The synaesthetes had either coloured letters, numbers, weekdays, or music, and the assumption was that these individuals might form a similar-enough group of synaesthesias to share the same genetic cause. Each person gave a sample of DNA, either from a blood sample in the early stages of the project, or later from a buccal swab (a sample taken by wiping something like a cotton-bud against the inside of the cheek). This DNA then underwent *whole-genome amplification* which produces larger samples of DNA from minute quantities. When the samples were analysed, the study provided evidence linking specific areas of the genome to synaesthesia. There was evidence that these families' synaesthesia was linked to chromosome 2 near a region known as 2a24. A subsequent study headed by Steffie Thomson and David Eagleman looked at a group with partially overlapping synaesthesias (coloured letters, numbers, weekdays, and months) and suggested a possible role for chromosome 16 (near 16q12.2-23.1) at least in some families.

The linkage studies above gave important early evidence for the role of genetics, but the regions identified contain hundreds of genes, and spanned hundreds of thousands of bases. One recent study has probed further into the genetics of synaesthesia to give pointers to specific genes. We talked above about the power of whole-genome sequencing but a cheaper and more efficient approach to DNA sequencing is to look only at the *exome*. The exome is a smaller part of the genome that happens to contain all the protein-coding genes. Since most genetic conditions can be traced back to these genes in particular, examining the exome is a useful starting point. The recent exome sequencing study looked again at three of the families with synaesthesia from the earlier family-linkage study of Asher and colleagues. These three families in particular had the same synaesthetic variant (sound-colour synaesthesia) affecting multiple family members over three or more generations. An exome sequencing approach found thirty-seven genes of interest, although none shared across all three families. Together then, the studies above suggest a divergence in the genetics of synaesthesia, where different forms of synaesthesia may be linked to different genes, and indeed, where different genes for the same synaesthetic variant may be at work in different families. We look closer at this now.

Knowing exactly which genes play a role in synaesthesia will be hampered by several important considerations. First, synaesthesia could involve important interactions between genes and the environment. This means that having the appropriate genetic make-up might not be enough to develop synaesthesia, and cases of discordant monozygotic twins (identical twins where only one experiences synaesthesia) support this contention. Another obvious example is that letter-colour synaesthesia is unlikely to develop without exposure to writing in early life. The same child raised in either a literate or non-literate society is likely to develop distinct types of synaesthesia: grapheme-colour synaesthesia in the former context (i.e. coloured letters) but, say, face-colour synaesthesia in the latter (i.e. colour when looking at faces; and I speculate face-colour synaesthesia because the region of the brain that processes letters in literate people appears to fire up for faces in non-literate individuals). So the same genetic code might give rise to different subtypes of synaesthesia. But it is also possible for different genetic codes to give rise to the same subtypes. In genetics this is known as *genetic heterogeneity*, where different genes produce the same phenotype which means the same outward manifestation.

Related to this complicated picture, we simply do not know whether synaesthesia is a single condition with a common genetic cause shared by all synaesthetes, or just an umbrella term for a group of genetically different conditions which nonetheless look behaviourally similar. There is some evidence both ways. Evidence for a shared genetic make-up across different types of synaesthesias comes from the fact that members of the same family can experience different forms of synaesthesia: a mother can give birth to a synaesthetic daughter whose words have colours but a synaesthetic son whose words have tastes. On the other hand, a hugely important study by Scott Novich, David Eagleman, and their collaborators in 2011 showed that subtypes of synaesthesias appear to occur in clusters. In their study, they examined over 12,000 synaesthetes, and found that certain synaesthesias clustered together: for example, people with number-colour synaesthesia were likely to have day-colour synaesthesia at above-chance levels, but were *no more* likely than the average person to have vision-smell synaesthesia. So coloured numbers and days were expressed together—along with coloured letters, months, and other sequences—in a single cluster. The researchers found five different clusters suggesting that some synaesthesias are likely to be expressed together so may have a shared genetic cause. In turn these may be distinct from the genetic origins of other types of synaesthesia. This fact, and the considerations above tell us that what stands before us is a considerable challenge when trying to link differences in the human genome to the different experiences of synaesthetes.

But once we start to fully understand the genetic make-up of people with synaesthesia, what might this actually tell us? What could the gene(s) responsible for synaesthesia actually do, and how might they give rise to the experiences of synaesthesia? In truth we have only very early ideas about which genes are involved, what proteins these genes might encode for, and what these proteins might ultimately do. But we saw in Chapter 2 that people with synaesthesia have differences in the way their brains are structured, so we might safely assume that genetic differences could play a role in creating these differences. Among the genes identified in the exome sequencing study described above, six genes in particular play a role in the formation of adult brain tissue (*SLIT2*, *MYO10*, *ROBO3*, *ITGA2*, *COL4A1*, and *SLC9A6*) and might therefore be implicated in the particular brain connectivity we have seen in adult synaesthetes. Elsewhere, neuroscientists Gary Bargary and Kevin Mitchell have suggested that any synaesthesia gene(s) could cause this 'cortical hyper-connectivity' in one of three broad ways. The first possible brain process is tied to genes that develop and guide axons. Remember that an axon is the long projection from each of the brain's neurons (nerve cells) which reaches out to other neurons to transmit electrical impulses. This establishes the connectivity between cortical areas, meaning that genes involved in how these axons are guided are therefore obvious candidates for playing a role in the brain architecture hypothesized in synaesthetes. Indeed a number of the core genes identified by the exome sequencing study above served this purpose. A second process which might be implicated in the genetic differences of synaesthetes is one that sets boundaries between different regions of the cortex and establishes barriers to axons trying to cross them. One final function which might play a role in developing synaesthesia is known as *synaptic pruning* or *apoptosis*. This is a natural process of cell death which eliminates synapses and takes place naturally within the developing brains of infants and children. This pre-programmed cell death lies at the heart of one of the most influential neurodevelopmental accounts of synaesthesia, which we turn to in more detail below.

Synaptic pruning and the Neonatal Synaesthesia Hypothesis

The *Neonatal* or *Infantile Synaesthesia Hypothesis* was originally proposed by psychologist Daphne Maurer and colleagues, and has captured the imagination of the research community with its elegant account of how synaesthesia might emerge in some people but not others. The theory rests on the notion of synaptic pruning. To understand synaptic pruning we must understand that an enormous number of connections in the brain are designed—surprisingly—to be transient. In other words they are designed to slowly die off during the course of normal childhood development. This means that the brains of babies have a larger number of connections compared to the brains of adults, and these connections are slowly pruned away as children grow up. But if normal pruning were disrupted in some people, hypothetically speaking, their adult brains might retain the high degree of connectivity from infancy, and would therefore have more abundant connections when compared to the average adult. This is the Neonatal Synaesthesia Hypothesis. In a nutshell it proposes that *all human infants are born as synaesthetes with hyper-connected brains* but that most people lose this ability during childhood via normal synaptic pruning (becoming adult non-synaesthetes) while a small number retain this ability because their synaptic pruning fails (becoming adult synaesthetes).

This hypothesis has been highly influential, appealing to scientists because it offers an elegant account for several observable facts about synaesthesia. These facts seem superficially different but can be united as the natural outcomes of this one theory. The first observation is that the human brain does indeed shows an extraordinary degree of connectivity during infancy with peak synaptic density just after birth. And we also saw in Chapter 2 that abundant neural connectivity is found in the brains of adult synaesthetes. So heightened connectivity relates to synaesthetic sensations, and is a feature of both adult synaesthetes and *all* babies. Along with this abundance of connectivity, there is evidence that babies have greater interplay between the senses. Infant brains show less specialization and segregation of sensory regions. For example, regions of the brain that usually respond to the *sounds* of language in adults respond to visual stimuli in 2-month-old babies. And related to this, there is evidence of direct anatomical connections during infancy from the auditory regions of the brain to the visual regions, with these particular connections greatly reduced or even absent in average adults.

Other support for the Neonatal Synaesthesia Hypothesis comes from a specific prediction that, if all people developed from the same infantile state, there might be similarities between adult synaesthetes and all other adults. Specifically, there may be tiny remnants of synaesthesia in all people, and if so, this 'shadow' of synaesthesia should mirror—albeit faintly—the overt, conscious experiences of true synaesthetes. Above we saw that some synaesthetic experiences do indeed mirror the intuitive cross-modal correspondences felt by all people. This has led some psychologists such as Gail Martino and Lawrence Marks to refer to non-synaesthetes' intuitive cross-modal correspondences as 'weak synaesthesia'. Finally, the neonatal hypothesis predicts that synaesthetic associations die out over time in most people, suggesting that children might show correspondences that adults no longer have. My study in Edinburgh of colourful touch showed exactly that. Our subjects were everyday people with cross-modal preferences to link smooth texture with light and vibrant colours, and our test-subjects ranged from 5 to 74 years of age. Most intriguingly, the association between smoothness and colour-vibrancy was found specifically in the younger subjects, but not in the older ones. This suggests that correspondences may indeed be dying out over time, just as the neonatal hypothesis would predict.

The Neonatal Synaesthesia Hypothesis is an elegant theory but it is not without its detractors. In Chapter 6 we will see arguments against the theory and look, too, at other controversies and outstanding issues facing the field. But here we have seen that synaesthesia emerges over time, and that it can follow rules based on information absorbed from the environment, with these rules sometimes shared by non-synaesthetes. We have seen that synaesthesia has a likely genetic inheritance. We can conclude therefore that synaesthesia derives not only from post-birth events such as literacy acquisition and environmental submersion, but is also likely to be predetermined in some way at birth.

Chapter 6
The question of synaesthesia

We will end our examination of synaesthesia by looking at areas of debate that are not yet fully resolved. I will speak about some of the unanswered questions—and indeed controversies, because of course scientists do not always agree. In the remaining pages of this book I will revisit some of the assumptions already discussed to show differing viewpoints and another side to these debates. And there are also many gaps in our knowledge. For example, we saw in Chapter 5 that synaesthesia is influenced by the environment, but most studies conducted have been on synaesthetes from an *English-speaking* environment. Just a few notable exceptions have looked at synaesthesia in speakers of Chinese, Japanese, Irish Gaelic, French, Czech, Dutch, Arabic, German, Swiss German, Spanish, Korean, Russian, and Greek. The findings in these studies have tended to reflect what we already know from studies on English speakers—that there is some degree of underlying structure to synaesthesia which sometimes reflects the language or environment synaesthetes are immersed in. Although this seems like a good start, we are still a long way from any kind of balance between understanding the synaesthetes in English-speaking cultures, and understanding synaesthetes worldwide. And a similar imbalance exists among different types of synaesthesias. I have looked in this book mostly at synaesthesias triggering colour, and synaesthesias triggered by language. Although these make up the majority of known synaesthesias, the experiences of other synaesthetes are just as valid and just as remarkable, even if they are less well-understood.

The Neonatal Synaesthesia Hypothesis revisited

One thing I have learned from researching synaesthesia is that the scientists working in this field happen to be a nice bunch. Conferences on synaesthesia are particularly welcoming and their academics are particularly agreeable. But of course people still sometimes disagree. And one area where they have strongly disagreed is in relation to the Neonatal Synaesthesia Hypothesis. We saw at the end of Chapter 5 that this hypothesis seeks to explain how synaesthesia develops from birth to adulthood. The theory notes that average babies and adult synaesthetes both have hyper-connected brains suggesting *all* babies may have synaesthesia, and that adult synaesthetes may simply fail to 'prune' the dense synaptic pathways we all had as babies.

The Neonatal Synaesthesia Hypothesis is an attractive theory because it pulls together several strands of evidence into a coherent whole, and it is rooted in a plausible account of brain development. However, it is a controversial theory which has drawn robust criticism from some quarters. First, any evidence for the theory is indirect and it remains on the whole untested. Neuro-imaging techniques have simply not yet been applied to the developing brains of baby synaesthetes. This means there is no direct evidence of whether their neural pathways fail to prune, or otherwise. And this is partly because it is not (yet) possible to diagnose synaesthesia in babies, although there might be ways around this. By brain scanning the offspring of adult synaesthetes we could observe their neurological development in the knowledge that these are the babies most likely to emerge as adult synaesthetes. But the practical limitations of this type of testing mean it has not yet been done. So there is no direct evidence for the Neonatal Theory in any longitudinal neuroscientific sense.

Other controversies for the theory relate to how we might interpret the cross-modal correspondences of all people. The Neonatal Theory predicts that adult non-synaesthetes should show 'weak synaesthesia' as some kind of remnant of their infantile synaesthetic past. And we saw in Chapter 5 that average people do indeed have synaesthesia-like associations across the senses or different modalities. We call these associations cross-modal correspondences. These correspondences are intuitive notions about the colours of sounds, the sounds of shapes, the textures of colours, and so on, which all people share at an unconscious level. And importantly they sometimes reflect the conscious experiences of synaesthetes (e.g. pairing high-pitch sounds with lighter rather than darker colours). But psychologists such as Orphelia Deroy and Charles Spence have suggested that cross-modal correspondences are irrelevant to the debate. They disagree with the idea that canonical conscious synaesthesia and general unconscious cross-modal correspondences are comparable enough to be considered continuous. They believe that similarities are only superficial and that placing weight on them means making unacceptable concessions to our models. So Deroy and Spence place low importance on the fact that similar rules operate across true synaesthesia and correspondences (e.g. high pitch mapping to lighter colours) and instead emphasize the notable differences. So unlike true synaesthesia, Deroy and Spence argue that correspondences are (a) pervasive rather than rare, (b) unconscious rather than conscious, (c) relative rather than absolute, (d) widely shared across non-synaesthetes (vs. more idiosyncratic in synaesthetes), and (e) transparent rather than obscure. The first two differences we have met already, but the remaining differences are as follows. In point (c) Deroy and Spence are noting that synaesthetes have specific concurrents (e.g. a certain shade of green for the piano note middle C) while a non-synaesthete has no single colour in mind (even if he or she prefers lighter colours for higher pitches). And, in points (d) and (e), Deroy and Spence are suggesting that non-synaesthetic correspondences are similar from one person to the next (e.g. that loud sound is felt to be large in size) while synaesthetes tend to differ between each other; and relatedly, that the associations of synaesthetes are more chaotic and illogical while the correspondences of non-synaesthetes can be easily traced to the environment (e.g. loud is large perhaps because large animals bellow while small ones squeak).

This might seem like a considerable weight of counter-evidence from Deroy and Spence, but controversy arises because certain scientists dispute their facts, and I would probably fall into this camp myself. On the whole, my own research has provided evidence *against* the 'idiosyncratic' notion of synaesthesia as a chaotic system with obscure roots (points (d) and (e) above). Instead, I and other colleagues have provided empirical evidence showing numerous ways in which the architecture that underlies synaesthesia is similar from one synaesthete to the next; how it is similar between synaesthetes and non-synaesthetes; and how it can even mirror the environment. This evidence is described in Chapter 5. But I suppose it is a matter of viewpoint. Where I see the similarities, Deroy and Spence see the differences. Where I see the bonds that unite synaesthetes and non-synaesthetes, they see the gaps that divide them. And there are indeed bonds, and there are indeed gaps.

Although I have questioned points (d) and (e), I agree fully with points (a), (b), and (c), which seem highly sensible to me. But these differences raised by Deroy and Spence have never been in doubt, and do not seem to challenge the neonatal hypothesis in my own mind. To me their argument appears to be that correspondences are not 'weak synaesthesia' because they are not strong synaesthesia. In other words, Deroy and Spence suggest there is no relationship between synaesthesia and correspondences because they are not identical, and I question this logic. Yes there are differences—because non-synaesthetes are not synaesthetes—but to say that they are entirely unrelated is to ignore their similarities. Deroy and Spence acknowledge these similarities (that neonates show sensory confusion; that adults have cross-modal correspondences; and that some correspondences follow rules found in synaesthesia) but propose that synaesthesia still arises from an entirely different pattern of development. In contrast, I would suggest that synaesthesia and correspondences show similarities at levels that are greater than chance so we might try to understand how those similarities came about. The Neonatal Synaesthesia Hypothesis is just one way to capture this. It may yet be flawed in other ways, but it cannot be rejected simply because synaesthetes and non-synaesthetes are not identical. So the pros and cons of the Neonatal Synaesthesia Hypothesis continue to divide the field. Although I find myself clearly on one side of the fence, I want to leave the reader in no doubt that both sides have their supporters, and that the field is firmly split on this issue—at least for now.

Consistency over time, revisited

In the opening pages of this book I laid out the key defining characteristics of synaesthesia. We saw that synaesthesia affects a small percentage of the population, who report extraordinary sensations of colours, tastes, shapes, etc., triggered by everyday activities such as reading, listening to music, eating, and so on. And among these defining features was that synaesthetic associations are consistent over time. For example, if the number 7 is forest green for any particular synaesthete, we have said it would be consistently forest green when the synaesthete is asked on repeated occasions. This characteristic been described in almost every science paper in the modern synaesthesia literature because convention states that synaesthetes *must*—by definition—be consistent in order to become test-subjects in our science studies. And this is because any person could pair a colour with a letter, or a shape with a taste, or a word with a flavour. But only synaesthetes have fixed unchanging associations. But in this section I will modify this claim in two ways. First, I will clarify that although synaesthetes are *highly* consistent, they are not necessarily 100 per cent consistent. But more importantly, we will also ask whether some synaesthetes might not be consistent at all.

So let's start with an uncontroversial clarification. Although synaesthetes who are test-subjects in psychology studies are highly consistent, they are not necessarily 100 per cent consistent. For example, the grapheme-colour synaesthetes in a study I ran in 2006 had consistency scores that ranged from 73 to 100 per cent, and this is typical. All were considered as synaesthetes because—importantly—they were all significantly more consistent than non-synaesthete control subjects. This much is uncontroversial, but is consistency actually necessary at all? Are there, in fact, genuine but *in*consistent synaesthetes? Received wisdom would say not; synaesthetes are included as test-subjects in scientific studies only after they pass a consistency test, meaning that virtually all synaesthetes reported in the literature are precisely those who show consistency. This approach allows us to rule out any people who claim to have synaesthesia falsely or in error. But one important drawback in using consistency in our central diagnostic for synaesthesia is the possibility that consistency is not a defining feature of synaesthesia at all. Or more specifically, it might be the defining features for most synaesthetes, but perhaps not all. I have encountered a small minority of individuals who appeared to understand what synaesthesia is, and who feel strongly that they experience it, and do not change their mind at a later date, but are not particularly consistent. So might consistency *not* be crucial to synaesthesia after all? Might it simply be a trait of some synaesthetes but not others?

This raises a number of intriguing questions, and perhaps the possibility that we are falling foul of a common scientific mistake called *Marslow's Law of the Instrument*. Psychologist Abraham Marslow famously stated that if the only tool we have is a hammer, there is a temptation to treat everything as if it were a nail. So although many synaesthetes *are* consistent, and although we have a tool that will assess consistency, our approach in rejecting self-declared synaesthetes that fail in consistency risks possibly overlooking genuine cases. And so I end this section with the following questions: Is synaesthesia truly consistent over time as a definitional criterion, or does consistency over time merely characterize a subset of synaesthetes? Have we been self-selecting a biased sample of consistent synaesthetes, while at the same time claiming that consistency is a necessary feature? And if so, is this 'consistency cornerstone' of modern synaesthesia research entirely circular? My own thoughts are that consistency is one useful feature to separate most synaesthetes from those who do not have synaesthesia. I think, too, that consistency is such a useful feature that we will rely on it to identify synaesthetes for many years to come. But I would also like to know whether some genuine synaesthesia can be fluid in certain individuals, and if so, what else makes these synaesthetes different to the rest.

The self-referral bias

All the studies I have described in this book were carefully planned and carried out with scientific expertise and presented in peer-reviewed journals, which means we can have a confidence in the results they produced. But in synaesthesia studies in particular, we have one particular problem which turns up time and time again, and which is relatively hard to mitigate against. It all comes down to the fact that synaesthesia is a rare condition. This means I cannot just open my door at the university and tap someone on the shoulder expecting him or her to be a synaesthete. And this in turn makes it relatively difficult to recruit test-subjects to take part in my synaesthesia studies, because I would have to do a lot of shoulder-tapping to find what could be deemed an acceptable number of synaesthetes to start running my study. Usually we would want at least thirty synaesthetes in any study group, and we would also want them to have the same type of synaesthesia to each other, just in case different synaesthetes behave in different ways. So if we were looking for grapheme-colour synaesthetes (found in around 1.5 per cent of the population),

I would have to tap 2,000 shoulders to find thirty synaesthetes. And assuming, say, one in five was even interested in taking part in my research, I would be tapping 10,000 shoulders to find enough people, even for a single study.

So, to save all that shoulder-tapping, psychologists post adverts, sometimes on the internet, or we take on media engagements where we describe our research to journalists who write articles (on the front page of, say, the *New York Times* if we are lucky). And then we get a very welcome deluge of emails from synaesthetes who recognized themselves in the story. All this is very good. Over the last seventeen years, my colleague, Jamie Ward, and I have been lucky enough to be contacted by thousands of people with synaesthesia, many of them offering to take part in our research. But what type of person reaches out to a scientist to offer to take part in science studies? In my mind they are of course a very welcome person indeed, but it is reasonable to expect they may have certain traits that make them different from the average person. For example, it is reasonable to assume they might be driven by intellectual curiosity, and may be the type of person who is open to the new experience of taking part in a science study. And therein lies the problem. When our study participants are recruited in such a way that they are likely to be high on certain traits anyway (e.g. Openness to Experience in their personality profile; see Chapter 4) we cannot conclude that such traits are typical of synaesthetes in general. We can only conclude that they are typical of the people who volunteered to take part in our study. Happily, synaesthesia studies have, on the whole, tried to use unbiased methods to recruit synaesthetes, and, crucially, recruitment is matched across synaesthetes and control groups. So where we looked at the personality traits of synaesthetes in Chapter 4 and found them high in the trait of Openness to Experience, we might be reasonably confident it is not due to the way they were recruited. But recruitment biases are always a risk and we should be ever-vigilant for them.

The politics of synaesthesia

In this book I have been minding my language. I have thought
carefully about the words I have used, not just so they might be
clear to the reader, but also that they may be politically sensitive.
Groups of synaesthetes have sprung up on the internet in the last
decade, and all have a valid voice to be heard. I have tried my
best to describe synaesthesia as a scientist who has probably spent
more time studying this phenomenon than most people on the
planet. But as a non-synaesthete I am only ever an observer. And
this is true even though I have seen synaesthesia up close in the
thousands of cases I have studied, and synaesthetes I have spoken to
face to face, or on the phone, or in letters and emails. And I have
even found synaesthesia close to home: sixteen years ago my
mother asked what new research I was working on and I told her
I was studying a group of people who think that, say, Tuesdays
are yellow. Without hesitation she declared 'Well everyone knows
Tuesdays are grey with a tweed texture'. I have since found
synaesthesia popping up throughout my family tree but I myself
am a non-synaesthete, and so I have offered a view of the science
literature from that vantage point.

But I have been careful in the language I have used. As a research
community, scientists tend to describe synaesthesia as a 'condition'.
It has been this way since we made an effort to change the earlier
unhealthy practice of describing synaesthesia as an 'abnormality',
or suggesting synaesthetes are different to 'normal' people.
Scientists describe synaesthesia as a condition because they are
looking for a word that does not imply illness or disease, but
which nonetheless reflects the fact that most people do not have
synaesthesia. I once met a synaesthete who disliked the term
'condition' because she wondered if it implies a need to cure.
But scientists who use this term do not want to imply this at
all—they are simply looking for as neutral a term as possible.
And we as a scientific community would be happy to adopt

another single-word noun that captures 'difference' without 'disease', if one were proposed. Perhaps we could think of synaesthesia as a 'trait' but what kind of trait might it be? It is not a personality trait, or a physical trait, but rather a trait of perception. But does the word 'trait' capture the fact that there might be co-morbidities (i.e. related health conditions) with synaesthesia such as higher rates of anxiety disorder? Does it capture the fact that a small number of synaesthetes are sometimes debilitated by the continuous bombardment of their senses—even if most are not? Does it capture that there are sometimes unwanted hyper-sensitivities—even alongside the joyful aspects of sensory creativity? Does it capture that while most children with synaesthesia are oblivious of their differences, others (with 'mirror-touch' synaesthesia) are feeling the physical pain of others? And does it capture the fact that I am contacted regularly by educational psychologists with a need to better understand how synaesthesia is contributing to the sensory difficulties of their child clients with autism? I simply do not know. Perhaps it does, and maybe we should adopt it. But I think it is important to heed the voices of people with synaesthesia in whichever direction that leads us—to balance out the need for accuracy with a desire for sensitivity.

Conclusions

This book provides an overview of synaesthesia as a snapshot of the field of research. We have seen a complex picture of how synaesthesia manifests itself, and what might cause it in terms of development, genetics, environment, and brain differences. And we have seen how it links to other traits such as improved memory or creativity in the arts. And we have seen that although synaesthesia seems superficially remarkable, it is a normal and perfectly expected outcome of how the brain extracts its sensory reality from the world around it. So this book is a reflection of the contemporary academic literature, which I hope will improve understanding of this remarkable phenomenon. I have spent many years at conferences, in lecture theatres, and in public places, describing synaesthesia to as many people as I can. But all the while that I have been describing synaesthetes as a group I have also been acknowledging that synaesthetes are individuals. All the while that I have been describing their differences from the average person, I have been acknowledging they form part of normal variations in the population. I have spoken to countless synaesthetes and reassured large numbers of parents who have contacted me, initially baffled by their children's descriptions of synaesthesia, and then relieved to know this is all perfectly normal and well-understood by science.

As I write the final words in this book I am stuck by what we do not yet understand about synaesthesia, but I am in awe of what we have been able to learn. If we look closely, we can find important facts about synaesthesia scattered among the pages of early science written in the 19th century. But as we saw in Chapter 1, much of what we know about synaesthesia today arose from a chance conversation between a man and his neighbour over dinner in 1980. Dr Richard Cytowic was innovative enough to take his neighbour's anecdotal account of synaesthesia and turn it into science. Others followed suit. Soon, neuroscientists had inspected the brains of synaesthetes; geneticists had examined their DNA; and psychologists had begun trying to understand how synaesthesia could develop and whether it is the same or different to cross-modal correspondences. Historians had begun uncovering its scientific past, while artists have been exploiting its beauty. A range of cognitive scientists have been homing in on its core properties by speaking to thousands of synaesthetes. And synaesthetes themselves have been moving all this forward with their generous willingness to take part in science studies. Together scientists, artists, and synaesthetes have drawn a fascinating picture. And the more I understand about this remarkable feature of the human mind, the more I would like to understand it better and to share this knowledge with the people who experience it.

Further reading and references

Chapter 1: What is synaesthesia?

'persons who have the tendency to use mental pictures…' Galton, F.
(1880). Visualised numerals. *Nature*, 21, 494.

'Madame L. has always personified numbers…' Flournoy, T. (1893).
Des phénomènes de synopsie, trans. J. Simner & E.M. Hubbard.
Paris: Felix Alcan, pp. 219–20.

'anyone expecting that such…' Duffy, P. L. (2002). *Blue Cats
and Chartreuse Kittens: How synesthetes color their worlds*.
New York: Times Books.

Cytowic, R. E. (2003). *The Man Who Tasted Shapes*. Cambridge,
MA: MIT Press.

Dixon, M. J., Smilek, D., & Merikle, P. M. (2004). Not all synaesthetes
are created equal: projector versus associator synaesthetes.
Cognitive, Affective & Behavioral Neuroscience, 4(3), 335–43.
Retrieved from http://www.ncbi.nlm.nih.gov/pubmed/15535169.

Duffy, P. L. (2002). *Blue Cats and Chartreuse Kittens: How synesthetes
color their worlds*. New York: Times Books.

Fassnidge, C. J., & Freeman, E. D. (2018). Sounds from seeing
silent motion: who hears them, and what looks loudest? *Cortex*.
http://doi.org/10.1016/j.cortex.2018.02.019.

Flournoy, T. (1893). *Des phénomènes de synopsie*. Paris: Felix Alcan.

Galton, F. (1880). Visualised numerals. *Nature*, 21, 494–5.

Plassart, A., & White, R. C. (2017). Théodore Flournoy on synesthetic
personification. *Journal of the History of the Neurosciences*, 26(1),
1–14. http://doi.org/10.1080/0964704X.2015.1077542.

Simner, J. (2007). Beyond perception: synaesthesia as a psycholinguistic phenomenon. *Trends in Cognitive Sciences*, 11(1). http://doi.org/10.1016/j.tics.2006.10.010.

Simner, J., & Carmichael, D. A. (2015). Is synaesthesia a dominantly female trait? *Cognitive Neuroscience*, 6(2–3), 68–76. http://doi.org/10.1080/17588928.2015.1019441.

Simner, J., & Hubbard, E. M. (2013). *The Oxford Handbook of Synesthesia*. Oxford: Oxford University Press.

Simner, J., Mulvenna, C., Sagiv, N., et al. (2006). Synaesthesia: the prevalence of atypical cross-modal experiences. *Perception*, 35(8). http://doi.org/10.1068/p5469.

Ward, J. (2008). *The Frog Who Croaked Blue: Synesthesia and the mixing of the senses*. London: Routledge.

Ward, J. (2013). Synesthesia. *Annual Review of Psychology*, 64(1), 49–75. http://doi.org/10.1146/annurev-psych-113011-143840.

Ward, J., Ipser, A., Phanvanova, E., Brown, P., Bunte, I., & Simner, J. (2018). The prevalence and cognitive profile of sequence-space synaesthesia. *Consciousness and Cognition*, 61. http://doi.org/10.1016/j.concog.2018.03.012.

Watson, D., Clark, L. A., & Tellegen, A. (1988). Development and validation of brief measures of positive and negative affect: The PANAS scales—University of Sussex. *Journal of Personality and Social Psychology*, 54(6), 1063–70.

Yong, Z., Hsieh, P.-J., & Milea, D. (2017). Seeing the sound after visual loss: functional MRI in acquired auditory-visual synesthesia. *Experimental Brain Research*, 235(2), 415–20. http://doi.org/10.1007/s00221-016-4802-6.

Chapter 2: Synaesthesia in the brain

'not in the eye but in the sensorium' Cooper, W.W. (1852). Vision. In R.B. Todd (ed.), In *The Cyclopædia of Anatomy and Physiology*, vol. 4/2. London: Longman, p. 1462.

'It was particularly striking [after ingesting LSD]...' Hollister, L. E. (1968). *Chemical Psychoses: LSD and Related Drugs*. Springfield, IL: Charles C. Thomas, p. 34.

Bargary, G., & Mitchell, K. J. (2008). Synaesthesia and cortical connectivity. *Trends in Neurosciences*. http://doi.org/10.1016/j.tins.2008.03.007.

Brang, D., & Ramachandran, V. S. (2008). Psychopharmacology of synesthesia: the role of serotonin S2a receptor activation. *Medical Hypotheses*. http://doi.org/10.1016/j.mehy.2007.09.007.

Cooper, W. W. (1852). Vision. In R.B. Todd (ed.), In *The Cyclopædia of Anatomy and Physiology*, vol. 4/2. London: Longman.

Hanggi, J., Wotruba, D., & Jancke, L. (2011). Globally altered structural brain network topology in grapheme-color synesthesia. *Journal of Neuroscience*, 31(15), 5816–28. http://doi.org/10.1523/JNEUROSCI.0964-10.2011.

Hollister, L. E. (1968). *Chemical Psychoses: LSD and Related Drugs*. Springfield, IL: Charles C. Thomas.

Hubbard, E. M., Arman, A. C., Ramachandran, V. S., & Boynton, G. M. (2005). Individual differences among grapheme-color synesthetes: brain-behavior correlations. *Neuron*, 45(6), 975–85. http://doi.org/10.1016/j.neuron.2005.02.008.

Hupé, J.-M., & Dojat, M. (2015). A critical review of the neuroimaging literature on synesthesia. *Frontiers in Human Neuroscience*, 9. http://doi.org/10.3389/fnhum.2015.00103.

Rouw, R., Scholte, H. S., & Colizoli, O. (2011). Brain areas involved in synaesthesia: a review. *Journal of Neuropsychology*, 5, 214–42. DOI:10.1111/j.1748-6653.2011.02006.x.

Simner, J., Rehme, M. K., Carmichael, D. A., et al. (2016). Social responsiveness to inanimate entities: altered white matter in a 'social synaesthesia. *Neuropsychologia*, 91. http://doi.org/10.1016/j.neuropsychologia.2016.08.020.

Van Leeuwen, T. M., Petersson, K. M., & Hagoort, P. (2010). Synaesthetic colour in the brain: beyond colour areas. A functional magnetic resonance imaging study of synaesthetes and matched controls. *PLoS ONE*. http://doi.org/10.1371/journal.pone.0012074.

Ward, J. (2015). Cognitive neuroscience of synesthesia: introduction to the special issue. *Cognitive Neuroscience*, 6(2–3), 45–7. http://doi.org/10.1080/17588928.2015.1055238.

Chapter 3: Synaesthesia and the arts

'created by animator Samantha Moore for a study...' Ward, J., Moore, S., Thompson-Lake, D., Salih, S., and Beck, B. (2008). The aesthetic appeal of auditory-visual synaesthetic perceptions in people without synaesthesia. *Perception*, 37(8), p. 1285–96.

Cretien van Campen. (2013). Synesthesia in the visual arts. In J. Simner & E. M. Hubbard (eds.), *The Oxford Handbook of Synesthesia* (pp. 631–46). Oxford: Oxford University Press.

Duffy, P. L. (2013). Synesthesia in literature. In J. Simner & E. M. Hubbard (eds.), *The Oxford Handbook of Synesthesia* (pp. 647–70). Oxford: Oxford University Press.

Duffy, P. L., & Simner, J. (2010). Synaesthesia in fiction. *Cortex*, 46(2). http://doi.org/10.1016/j.cortex.2008.11.003.

Johnson, D., Allison, C., & Baron-Cohen, S. (2013). The prevalence of synesthesia: the consistency revolution. In J. Simner & E. M. Hubbard (eds.), *The Oxford Handbook of Synesthesia* (pp. 3–23). Oxford: Oxford University Press.

Rothen, N., & Meier, B. (2010). Higher prevalence of synaesthesia in art students. *Perception*, 39(5), 718–20. http://doi.org/10.1068/p6680.

Steen, C., & Berman, G. (2013). *Synesthesia and the Artistic Process*, ed. J. Simner & E. M. Hubbard. Oxford: Oxford University Press.

Ward, J., Moore, S., Thompson-Lake, D., Salih, S., & Beck, B. (2008). The aesthetic appeal of auditory-visual synaesthetic perceptions in people without synaesthesia. *Perception*, 37(8), 1285–96. http://doi.org/10.1068/p5815.

Chapter 4: Is synaesthesia a 'gift' or a 'condition'?

'Numbers are my friends...' Tammet, D. (2007). *Born On a Blue Day. Inside the Extraordinary Mind of an Autistic Savant: A Memoir*. New York: Free Press, p. 2.

Banissy, M. J., Tester, V., Muggleton, N. G., et al. (2013). Synesthesia for color is linked to improved color perception but reduced motion perception. *Psychological Science*, 24(12), 2390–7. http://doi.org/10.1177/0956797613492424.

Baron-Cohen, S., Johnson, D., Asher, J., et al. (2013). Is synaesthesia more common in autism? *Molecular Autism*, 4(1), 40. http://doi.org/10.1186/2040-2392-4-40.

Chun, C. A., & Hupé, J.-M. (2016). Are synesthetes exceptional beyond their synesthetic associations? A systematic comparison of creativity, personality, cognition, and mental imagery in synesthetes and controls. *British Journal of Psychology*, 107(3), 397–418. http://doi.org/10.1111/bjop.12146.

Derbyshire, S. W. G., Osborn, J., & Brown, S. (2013). Feeling the pain of others is associated with self-other confusion and prior pain

experience. *Frontiers in Human Neuroscience*, 7. http://doi.
org/10.3389/fnhum.2013.00470.

Hughes, J. E. A., Simner, J., Baron-Cohen, S., Treffert, D. A., & Ward,
J. (2017). Is synaesthesia more prevalent in autism spectrum
conditions? Only where there is prodigious talent. *Multisensory
Research*, 30(3–5). http://doi.org/10.1163/22134808-00002558.

Lacey, S., Martinez, M., McCormick, K., & Sathian, K. (2016).
Synesthesia strengthens sound-symbolic cross-modal
correspondences. *European Journal of Neuroscience*, 44(9),
2716–21. http://doi.org/10.1111/ejn.13381.

Medina, J., & DePasquale, C. (2017). Influence of the body schema on
mirror-touch synesthesia. *Cortex*, 88, 53–65. http://doi.
org/10.1016/j.cortex.2016.12.013.

Meier, B., & Rothen, N. (2013). Synesthesia and memory. In J. Simner
& E. M. Hubbard (eds.), *The Oxford Handbook of Synesthesia*
(pp. 692–707). Oxford: Oxford University Press.

Neufeld, J., Roy, M., Zapf, A., et al. (2013). Is synesthesia more
common in patients with Asperger syndrome? *Frontiers in Human
Neuroscience*, 7, 847. http://doi.org/10.3389/fnhum.2013.00847.

Simner, J., Ipser, A., Smees, R., & Alvarez, J. (2017). Does synaesthesia
age? Changes in the quality and consistency of synaesthetic
associations. *Neuropsychologia*, 106. http://doi.org/10.1016/j.
neuropsychologia.2017.09.013.

Speed, L. J., & Majid, A. (2018). Superior olfactory language and
cognition in odor-color synaesthesia. *Journal of Experimental
Psychology: Human perception and performance*, 44(3), 468–81.
http://doi.org/10.1037/xhp0000469.

Tammet, D. (2007). *Born On a Blue Day. Inside the Extraordinary
Mind of an Autistic Savant: A Memoir*. New York: Free Press.

Ward, J., Hoadley, C., Hughes, J. E. A., et al. (2017). Atypical sensory
sensitivity as a shared feature between synaesthesia and autism.
Scientific Reports, 7. http://doi.org/10.1038/srep41155.

Ward, J., Rothen, N., Chang, A., & Kanai, R. (2017). The structure
of inter-individual differences in visual ability: evidence from
the general population and synaesthesia. *Vision Research*, 141,
293–302. http://doi.org/10.1016/j.visres.2016.06.009.

Chapter 5: Where does synaesthesia come from?

Asher, J. E., Lamb, J. A., Brocklebank, D., et al. (2009).
A whole-genome scan and fine-mapping linkage study of

auditory-visual synesthesia reveals evidence of linkage to chromosomes 2q24, 5q33, 6p12, and 12p12. *The American Journal of Human Genetics*, 84(2), 279–85. http://doi.org/10.1016/j.ajhg.2009.01.012.

Kosslyn, S. M., Thompson, W. L., & Alpert, N. M. (1997). Neural systems shared by visual imagery and visual perception: a Positron Emission Tomography study. *NeuroImage*, 6(4), 320–34. http://doi.org/10.1006/NIMG.1997.0295.

Ludwig, V. U., & Simner, J. (2013). What colour does that feel? Tactile-visual mapping and the development of cross-modality. *Cortex*, 49(4). http://doi.org/10.1016/j.cortex.2012.04.004.

Mankin, J. L., & Simner, J. (2017). A is for apple: the role of letter-word associations in the development of grapheme-colour synaesthesia. *Multisensory Research*, 30(3–5). http://doi.org/10.1163/22134808-00002554.

Maurer, D., Gibson, L. C., & Spector, F. (2013). Synesthesia in infants and very young children. In J. Simner & E. M. Hubbard (eds.), *The Oxford Handbook of Synesthesia* (pp. 46–64). Oxford: Oxford University Press.

Newell, F. N., & Mitchell, K. J. (2016). Multisensory integration and cross-modal learning in synaesthesia: a unifying model. *Neuropsychologia*, 88, 140–50. http://doi.org/10.1016/j.neuropsychologia.2015.07.026.

Novich, S., Cheng, S., & Eagleman, D. M. (2011). Is synaesthesia one condition or many? A large-scale analysis reveals subgroups. *Journal of Neuropsychology*, 5(2), 353–71. http://doi.org/10.1111/j.1748-6653.2011.02015.x.

Simner, J., Ward, J., Lanz, M., et al. (2005). Non-random associations of graphemes to colours in synaesthetic and non-synaesthetic populations. *Cognitive Neuropsychology*, 22, 1069–85.

Tilot, A. K., Kucera, K. S., Vino, A., et al. (2018). Rare variants in axonogenesis genes connect three families with sound–color synesthesia. *Proceedings of the National Academy of Sciences*, 115(12), 3168–73. http://doi.org/10.1073/pnas.1715492115.

Tomson, S. N., Avidan, N., Lee, K., et al. (2011). The genetics of colored sequence synesthesia: suggestive evidence of linkage to 16q and genetic heterogeneity for the condition. *Behavioural Brain Research*, 223(1), 48–52. http://doi.org/10.1016/j.bbr.2011.03.071

Watson, M. R., Akins, K. A., Spiker, C., Crawford, L., & Enns, J. T. (2014). Synesthesia and learning: a critical review and novel theory. *Frontiers in Human Neuroscience*, 8, 98. http://doi. org/10.3389/fnhum.2014.00098.

Witthoft, N., Winawer, J., & Eagleman, D. M. (2015). Prevalence of learned grapheme-color pairings in a large online sample of synesthetes. *PLoS ONE*. http://doi.org/10.1371/journal. pone.0118996.

Chapter 6: The question of synaesthesia

Christensen, D. L., Baio, J., Braun, K. V. N., et al. (2016). Prevalence and characteristics of autism spectrum disorder among children aged 8 years: Autism and Developmental Disabilities Monitoring Network, 11 sites, United States, 2012. *Morbidity and Mortality Weekly Report: Surveillance summaries*, 65(3), 1–23. http://doi. org/10.15585/mmwr.ss6503a1.

Deroy, O., & Spence, C. (2013). Why we are not all synesthetes (not even weakly so). *Psychonomic Bulletin & Review*, 20(4), 643–64. http://doi.org/10.3758/s13423-013-0387-2.

Root, N. B., Rouw, R., Asano, M., et al. (2018). Why is the synesthete's 'A' red? Using a five-language dataset to disentangle the effects of shape, sound, semantics, and ordinality on inducer–concurrent relationships in grapheme-color synesthesia. *Cortex*, 99, 375–89. http://doi.org/10.1016/j.cortex.2017.12.003.

Simner, J. (2012). Defining synaesthesia. *British Journal of Psychology*, 103(1), 1–15. http://doi.org/10.1348/0007126 10X528305.

Simner, J. (2013). The 'rules' of synesthesia. In J. Simner & E. M. Hubbard (eds.), *The Oxford Handbook of Synesthesia* (pp. 149–65). Oxford: Oxford University Press.

Spector, F., & Maurer, D. (2009). Synesthesia: a new approach to understanding the development of perception. *Developmental Psychology*, 45(1), 175–89. http://doi.org/10.1037/a0014171.

Van Leeuwen, T. M., Trautmann-Lengsfeld, S. A., Wallace, M. T., Engel, A. K., & Murray, M. M. (2016). Bridging the gap: synaesthesia and multisensory processes. *Neuropsychologia*, 88, 1–4. http://doi.org/10.1016/j.neuropsychologia.2016.06.007.

Index

A

acquired synaesthesia *see* congenital vs acquired synaesthesia

advantages and disadvantages of synaesthesia 59–63

alphabet books 86, 88–9

animation 58–60

apoptosis 101–4

artistic process 43 *see also* Steen Carol, Layden, Timothy B., Söffing, Christine, Torke, Michael, Moore Samantha

Asperger's syndrome *see* autism-spectrum conditions (ASC)

associator and projector synaesthesia 5–6, 12–13, 37, 39–40

autism *see* autism-spectrum conditions (ASC)

autism spectrum conditions (ASC) 78–81, 113–14

Autism Spectrum Quotient 79–81

B

binding *see* hyperbinding

blindfolding 31–4 *see also* congenital vs acquired synaesthesia

blindness 31–2

brain-based models of synaesthesia 20–42

C

causes of synaesthesia *see* brain-based models of synaesthesia, genetics and inheritance, developmental origins

childhood synaesthesia 5–6, 18–19, 47–8, 74, 81, 88–90, 99–100, 102–3, 113–15

chromosomes 94–6, 98–9

Clouds Rise Up (Steen, 2004) 55–6

cognitive abilities (of synaesthetes) 13–14, 66–9

colour blindness 97

colour centre *see* visual cortex, colour processing

colour processing 28–30, 37, 41–2

coloured alphabet *see* grapheme-colour synaesthesia

coloured graphemes *see* grapheme-colour synaesthesia

coloured hearing *see* music-colour synaesthesia

coloured letters *see* grapheme-colour synaesthesia

coloured music *see* music-colour synaesthesia

coloured numbers *see* grapheme-colour synaesthesia

concurrent *see* inducer and concurrent

congenital vs acquired synaesthesia 18–19, 33 *see also* blindness, blindfolding

connectivity *see* white matter connectivity

consequences of synaesthesia *see* advantages and disadvantages

consistency testing 3–4, 51–5, 109–10

cortical connectivity *see* white matter connectivity

creativity (of synaesthetes) 43–66

cross-modal correspondences 72–4, 90–4, 107–9, 115

cross-modality 70–1

cross-talk *see* cross-activation

Cytowic, Richard 7–8, 24–5, 115

D

Dark Glistening (Layden, 2010) 56–7

Day, Sean 17–18, 49–50

definition, problems in defining 3–5, 8–9, 13–15, 18–19, 109–11

deoxyribonucleic acid (DNA) 83, 94–9, 115

diagnosing synaesthesia *see* test of genuineness

diffusion tensor imaging (DTI) 23–4, 34–41

digits *see* graphemes

disadvantages *see* advantages and disadvantages of synaesthesia

disinhibited feedback model 30–5, 37–9

DNA *see* deoxyribonucleic acid (DNA)

drug-induced synaesthesias *see* congenital vs. acquired Synaesthesia

E

eye 2–3, 21–4, 97

F

family-linkage studies 98–9 *see also* genetics and inheritance

feedback *see* disinhibited feedback model

female to male ratios *see* self-report biases

flavour 1–2, 7–8, 17–18, 52–4, 74–7, 83–4, 88, 90, 109–10 *see also* lexical-gustatory synaesthesia

fractional anisotropy (FA) *see* diffusion tensor imaging (DTI)

functional magnetic resonance imaging (fMRI) 23–4, 26–9, 31–2, 37–9, 41–2

G

Galton, Francis 9–12

gender bias *see* self-report biases

genetics and inheritance 5–6, 8, 16–17, 83, 114–15

graphemes (letters and numbers) 5–6, 8–17, 26–7, 30, 32–4, 37–41, 44–6, 51–4, 68–70, 81–91, 94, 98–101, 109–10, 113

grapheme-colour synaesthesia 13–14, 28–33, 37–42, 45–6, 66–9, 77–9, 81, 85, 88–91, 99–101, 110–12

grey matter 35–6, 38–9, 41, 67–8

H

hallucinogenic drugs *see* congenital vs. acquired synaesthesia

history of synaesthesia 9–12, 15–16, 23–4, 87–8, 115
hyperbinding 38–40
hyperconnectivity *see* white matter connectivity

I

imagery *see* mental imagery
inducer and concurrent 4–5, 8–9, 14–19, 37–40, 51–2, 69, 83–90

K

Kandinsky, Wassily 44–5

L

languages (other than English) 15, 71, 105–6
Layden, Timothy B. 56–9
letter-colour synaesthesia *see* grapheme-colour synaesthesia
lexical-gustatory synaesthesia 1–2, 52–4, 74–7, 88 *see also* flavor, Wanncrton, James lysergic acid diethylamide (LSD) *see* congenital vs. acquired synaesthesia

M

Man Who Tasted Shapes, The 7–8
mathematics 69–70, 81–2
memory 62, 65–70, 80–1, 114–15
mental imagery 5–6, 12, 28–30, 37, 39–40
Messiaen, Olivier 44–5
mind's eye *see* mental imagery
mirror-touch synaesthesia 74–5, 113–14
Moore, Samantha *see* animation
motion perception 66–8 *see also* motion-sound synaesthesia

motion-sound synaesthesia 2, 7–8, 33
music 3–6, 8–9, 18, 31–2, 43–7, 49–50, 55–60, 62–3, 91, 98–9, 109–10
music-colour synaesthesia *see* music, sound-colour synaesthesia

N

Nabokov, Vladimir 44–5
Neonatal Synaesthesia Hypothesis 102–4, 106–8
number-colour synaesthesia, *see* grapheme-colour synaesthesia
number lines *see* sequence-space synaesthesia

O

olfaction *see* smell
onomatopoeia *see* sound symbolism
ordinal linguistic personification (OLP) *see* sequence-personality synaesthesia
origin of term 'synaesthesia' 18–19

P

parietal cortex 22, 38–40, 75
Penfield, Wilder 22–3
perception 26, 33, 56–7, 62, 66–7
perceptual reality of synaesthetic colour 1–2, 5–6, 17–18
personification *see* sequence-personality synaesthesia
phoneme-colour synaesthesia 13–14
pi (mathematical constant) 81–2
Positron Emission Tomography (PET) 23–6, 28

prevalence 2, 8, 48–9, 111–12
projector synaesthesia
  see associator and projector
  synaesthesia
psilocybin *see* congenital vs.
  acquired synaesthesia

Q

Questionnaires (autism,
  personality, sensory
  sensitivities) 65–6, 78–9

R

re-entrant processing model 38–9
'rules' of synaesthesia 13–14, 84–90

S

savant syndrome 79–81
  see also Tammet, Daniel
seeing vs knowing 5–6
self-report biases 2, 33,
  44–9, 111–12
sensory deprivation *see* blindfolding
sequence-personality synaesthesia
  15–17, 40–1, 81, 87–8
sequence-space synaesthesia 8–15,
  33, 69–70, 91
serotonin *see* neurotransmitter
sex ratio *see* self-report biases
sign language 5–6
smell 2–4, 13–14, 17–18, 22–3,
  51–2, 100–1
Söffing, Christine 6–7, 56–7
sound-colour synaesthesia 4–9,
  18, 46–9, 91, 98–9, *see also*
  Day, Sean, Layden, Timothy B.,
  Söffing, Christine, Steen, Carol,
  Torke, Michael

sound-symbolism 71–3
Steen, Carol 55–6
strong vs weak synaesthesia 103–4,
  107–9
synaptic pruning *see* apoptosis

T

Tammet, Daniel 81–2 *see also*
  savant syndrome
taste *see* flavour
Test of Genuineness *see* consistency
  testing
textures 6–8, 54–6, 60, 78–9, 81
time-space synaesthesia
  see sequence-space synaesthesia
Torke, Michael 43, 50–1, 58
touch *see* mirror-touch
  synaesthesia, texture, *Man Who
  Tasted Shapes, The*, touch-colour
  synaesthesia
touch-colour synaesthesia 2, 87–8,
  91–4 *see also* blindness,
  blindfolding
Transcranial Magnetic Stimulation
  (TMS) 67–8

V

variants of synaesthesia 2–18
  see also grapheme-colour
  synaesthesia, sound-colour
  synaesthesia, sequence-space
  synaesthesia, sequence-
  personality synaesthesia,
  touch-colour synaesthesia,
  taste-shape synaesthesia
visual cortex 28–30, 37, 41–2
visuo-spatial synaesthesia
  see sequence-space
  synaesthesia

W

Wannerton, James 1–4, 17–18, 74–7

Watson, Michael 7–9

weak synaesthesia *see* strong vs weak synaesthesia

web communities 113

white matter connectivity 35–7, 40–1 *see also* diffusion tensor imaging

whole-genome amplification 98–9

word-taste synaesthesia *see* lexical-gustatory synaesthesia

Index

SOCIAL MEDIA
Very Short Introduction

Join our community

www.oup.com/vsi

- Join us online at the official Very Short Introductions **Facebook** page.
- Access the thoughts and musings of our authors with our online **blog**.
- Sign up for our monthly **e-newsletter** to receive information on all new titles publishing that month.
- Browse the full range of Very Short Introductions online.
- Read **extracts** from the Introductions for free.
- If you are a teacher or lecturer you can order inspection copies quickly and simply via our website.